Key Concepts in Arthroplasty

Key Concepts in Arthroplasty

Edited by **Robert Berry**

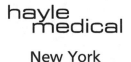

New York

Published by Hayle Medical,
30 West, 37th Street, Suite 612,
New York, NY 10018, USA
www.haylemedical.com

Key Concepts in Arthroplasty
Edited by Robert Berry

International Standard Book Number: 978-1-63241-272-0 (Hardback)

Printed in the United States of America.

Contents

Permissions

List of Contributors

Preface

This book was inspired by the evolution of our times; to answer the curiosity of inquisitive minds. Many developments have occurred across the globe in the recent past which has transformed the progress in the field.

Essential concepts of arthroplasty have been vividly presented in this book. Success of Sir Charnley's total hip arthroplasty has inspired many researchers to study this subject in detail and analyze its various aspects. Arthroplasty basically deals with joints of upper extremity and spine. However, any foreign design brought to the human body could lead to complications. The book discusses the topic of infections which includes complete analysis, detailed description and management of this difficult condition.

This book was developed from a mere concept to drafts to chapters and finally compiled together as a complete text to benefit the readers across all nations. To ensure the quality of the content we instilled two significant steps in our procedure. The first was to appoint an editorial team that would verify the data and statistics provided in the book and also select the most appropriate and valuable contributions from the plentiful contributions we received from authors worldwide. The next step was to appoint an expert of the topic as the Editor-in-Chief, who would head the project and finally make the necessary amendments and modifications to make the text reader-friendly. I was then commissioned to examine all the material to present the topics in the most comprehensible and productive format.

I would like to take this opportunity to thank all the contributing authors who were supportive enough to contribute their time and knowledge to this project. I also wish to convey my regards to my family who have been extremely supportive during the entire project.

Editor

Part 1

Infection

Infections in Hip and Knee Arthroplasty: Challenges to and Chances for the Microbiological Laboratory

Peter Schäfer[1], Bernd Fink[2], Dieter Sandow[1] and Lars Frommelt[3]
[1]MVZ Labor Ludwigsburg, Wernerstrasse 33, Ludwigsburg,
[2]Department of Joint Replacement, General and Rheumatic Orthopaedics,
Orthopaedic Clinic Markgröningen, Kurt-Lindemann-Weg 10, Markgröningen,
[3]Institute for Infectiology, ENDO-Clinic Hamburg, Holstenstrasse 2, Hamburg
Germany

1. Introduction

Comprehensive algorithms have been devised to improve the management of periprosthetic joint infections of the hip and the knee (Gomez & Patel, 2011a, 2011b; Peel et al., 2011). There is still no single best method for diagnosis, as stressed for instance in a guideline published recently by the American Association of Orthopedic Surgeons (AAOS) (Della Valle et al., 2010). An important reason for this is lacking consensus on how to define arthroplasty infection accurately. Nevertheless, it is beyond dispute that microbiologic techniques play a key role in assessment for these infections.

The chapter consists of three sections. Firstly, a general introduction to the special nature of arthroplasty infection is given, which highlights the necessity of reliable microbiological diagnostics. Secondly, a critical appraisal of the various technical and interpretive aspects of microbiologic procedures is featured. Thirdly, our own diagnostic approaches are presented, and a prospect on probable useful developments in the future is offered.

2. Identification of infected implants: The need for microbiological testing

2.1 Epidemiology

Periprosthetic joint infections are a feared complication of hip and knee arthroplasty. Infection is supposed to be the underlying cause in about 15% of hip revision arthroplasties and 25% of knee revision arthroplasties (Bozic et al., 2009, 2010). Depending on the onset of infection after the primary implantation, periprosthetic infections have been defined as "early" (up to 3 months), "delayed" (3-24 months), and "late" (more than 24 months) after surgery (Zimmerli et al., 2004). However, a different classification makes more sense from the therapeutic point of view. According to this, infections which occur within 4 weeks after arthroplasty implantation are recognized as "early". These are most often caused by highly virulent organisms (e. g. *Staphylococcus aureus*) acquired during or shortly after implantation and can be treated with the prospect of survival of the implant. In contrast, infections which become manifest after more than 4 weeks ("late" infections) require removal of the prosthesis. Late infections are low-grade infections due to less virulent agents belonging to the normal skin flora (e. g. coagulase-negative staphylococci, *Propionibacterium* species, coryneform bacteria), which are mostly also attained during the operation procedure or are infections which result from hematogenous spreading from remote sites (Cui et al., 2007; Hanssen & Osmon, 2002; Virolainen et al., 2002).

2.2 Pathogenetic aspects

The characteristics of arthroplasty infection reflect a unique pathogenesis which is ultimately marked by two features: biofilm development and manifestation of a periprosthetic membrane.

2.2.1 Biofilms

Biofilm-forming bacteria share the ability to colonize foreign implant materials by initial attachment to the surface, followed by agglomeration in multi-cellular layers. During the accumulation process the bacteria excrete matrix substances into which the infectious agents themselves become embedded. Due to alterations in cellular metabolism, regulated by complex signal pathways within the biofilm, the bacteria switch from the planktonic state to a sessile condition in which proliferation rates are extremely low (Costerton et al., 1999; Donlan & Costerton, 2002; Donlan, 2005; Gristina & Costerton, 1985).

Infections involving biofilm formation are both difficult to identify and to treat. On one hand, the biofilm matrix provides a substantial barrier to host defense mechanisms and to diffusion of antibiotics. On the other hand, the low proliferation levels of the sessile organisms may dramatically impair their antibiotic susceptibility, especially to bactericidal agents (Jones et al., 2001; Monzon et al., 2002; Stewart & Costerton, 2001), and their cultivation for diagnostic purposes in vitro.

As biofilm formation is a gradual process, this mechanism is the characteristic feature of late, low-grade infections. Implants with an established biofilm are definitely subject to removal although the causative agents are less virulent by themselves than the bacteria which cause early arthroplasty infections.

2.2.2 Periprosthetic membrane

The periprosthetic membrane is the histomorphologic hallmark of joint implant failure. It is a seam of connective tissue which develops at the interface between the bone and the implant in the course of the inflammatory process that leads to septic or aseptic prosthetic loosening. Interestingly, there are four morphologic types which can be linked to different etiologies of inflammation. Of these, the infectious type (type II) is particularly often associated with periprosthetic infection. It is characterized by predominant infiltration with neutrophilic polymorphonuclear leukocytes (Krenn et al., 2011; Morawietz et al., 2006).

As the periprosthetic membrane must be removed if the surgical revision procedure is to be successful, it is ideal sample material for characterizing the type of inflammation by histology, thus providing valuable evidence for the underlying cause of implant loosening.

2.3 Inflammation parameters: Utility to detect infections

Early periprosthetic infections are mostly associated with typical clinical signs of infectious disease. However, in low-grade (late) infections the clinical symptoms and radiologic signs are often unspecific and therefore not suitable for ruling out aseptic implant failure

(Virolainen et al., 2002). Nuclear imaging techniques used to detect periprosthetic inflammation are generally regarded as optional tests which may be of use if the diagnosis cannot be established otherwise, but they are not recommended for routine application (Della Valle et al., 2010). In contrast, the following procedures do play important roles in patient assessment for arthroplasty infection.

2.3.1 Blood laboratory markers
Erythrocyte sedimentation rate (ESR) and C-reactive protein (CRP) level are the parameters most widely used for preoperative evaluation of patients with suspected arthroplasty infection. While sensitivity is mostly high, specificity is limited, especially in patients with systemic inflammatory diseases (e. g., rheumatoid arthritis) (Bottner et al., 2007; Della Valle et al., 2007; Fink et al., 2008; Greidanus et al., 2007; Kamme & Lindberg, 1981). Nevertheless, from the studies with reliable data the AAOS strongly recommends testing of both ESR and CRP in all patients assessed for arthroplasty infection (Della Valle et al., 2010).
Other inflammation markers (interleukin 6, procalcitonin, tumor necrosis factor α) are evaluated increasingly for periprosthetic infections, but at present there seems to be no advantage over CRP testing (Berbari et al., 2010; Bottner et al., 2007; Di Cesare et al., 2005).

2.3.2 Microscopic detection of inflammatory cells
Joint aspiration fluid. Total and differential white blood cell counts in synovial fluid are routinely determined in many settings. Some studies of knee patients have reported that total leukocyte counts or neutrophils percentages which exceed a certain cutoff level are highly indicative of arthroplasty infection. However, the thresholds differ considerably between studies (Della Valle et al., 2007; Ghanem et al., 2008; Trampuz et al., 2004).
In contrast, there are less data available for hip patients because aspiration of this joint is more prone to complications and is therefore only recommended if there is substantial clinical or laboratory evidence for infection (Della Valle et al., 2010; Schinsky et al., 2008).
Frozen tissue sections. Neutrophils are the predominant histomorphologic factor in periprosthetic infection (Krenn et al., 2011; Morawietz et al., 2006). As a consequence, the histologic diagnosis of probable infections is based on the tissue neutrophil concentration, as defined by i) the number of neutrophils in a high-power (400x) microscopic field, and ii) the minimum number of fields (usually 10) containing that concentration of neutrophils. The available studies report 5 or 10 neutrophils per high-power field as suitable thresholds for diagnosis of arthroplasty infection (Banit et al., 2002; Della Valle et al., 2007; Fehring & McAlister, 1994; Fink et al., 2008; Frances Borrego et al., 2007; Ko et al., 2005; Lonner et al., 1996; Nunez et al., 2007; Schinsky et al., 2008). Patients with inflammatory arthropathy, which often display tissue infiltration by neutrophils in the absence of infection, were excluded in some of these investigations (Fehring & McAlister, 1994; Ko et al., 2005; Pandey et al., 1999; Schinsky et al., 2008). However, all in all there is not enough information to enable a clear-cut preference of the lower or the higher threshold.
Despite the considerable advances in recent years with respect to the histomorphologic characterization of periprosthetic infections, it is not possible to treat affected patients sufficiently unless the causative microorganisms are identified precisely. Thus, customized local and systemic antibiotic therapy of a known infectious agent is inherently superior to calculated therapy because treatment failure arising from antibiotic resistance can be avoided (Bejon et al., 2010).

3. Microbiological diagnosis: Pros and cons of different approaches

Adequate microbiological procedures must reflect the special character of periprosthetic infections in order to identify the causative agents accurately. Although largely interdependent, eight issues which may influence the significance of microbiologic testing are addressed separately in the following: i) patient-specific factors, ii) the sample character, iii) the logistic interface between the clinic and the laboratory, iv) the method of sample processing, v) the means of identification, vi) the culture conditions, vii) the means of discriminating between infection and contamination, and viii) the stage at which sample materials are drawn (pre-operatively versus intra-operatively).

3.1 Patient-specific factors
3.1.1 Sample origin (hip versus knee)
Joint aspiration prior to revision arthroplasty is widely utilized. For knee patients the procedure is comparatively straightforward, whereas hip aspiration may impose a higher risk of iatrogenic infection. Thus, it is often argued that invasive diagnostic samples from hip patients should be obtained only if a there is a high probability of infection (Bozic et al., 2009, 2010).
Regarding periprosthetic tissue biopsies, the diagnostic sensitivity of pre-operative sampling may be lower in hip infections compared with knee infections (Fink et al., 2008; Meermans & Haddad, 2010; Williams et al., 2004), possibly because infected tissue is more difficult to assess without dislocating the joint.

3.1.2 Underlying systemic diseases
The definitive identification of microorganisms is especially important in patients with systemic inflammatory diseases because, as mentioned before, inflammation markers can be elevated in aseptic implant failure. At the same time, the differentiation between an infecting and a contaminating agent is challenging in these patients (see 3.7).

3.1.3 Previous antibiotic therapy
False-negative results of microbiological cultures and even PCR tests have been reported in patients who received antibiotic therapy within 2 weeks prior to obtaining intra-articular sample material (Achermann et al., 2010). Furthermore, it is also suggested that peri-operative antibiotic prophylaxis should be withheld if possible until samples for microbiological analysis have been obtained, but that the risk of false-negative sample results also should be weighed against the protective effect of pre-operative administration of antibiotic prophylaxis (Achermann et al., 2010; Engesaeter et al., 2003; Jämsen et al., 2009; Trampuz et al., 2007).

3.2 Sample character
3.2.1 Tissue swabs
In a report on hip and knee patients organisms cultured from swabs of sinus tracts showed no concordance with the culture results from specimens obtained intra-operatively (Sadiq et al., 2005). There are limited data which suggest that the results of superficial swabs show a reasonable correlation with culture yield from intra-operative tissue biopsy material (Cune et al., 2009). However, other studies have rated results from swab material as both insensitive and unspecific (Font-Vizcarra et al., 2010; Levine & Evans, 2001). Swabs cannot

absorb nearly as much material as can be harvested from tissue biopsies or joint fluid, which alone would account for inferior sensitivity. Furthermore, as most etiologic agents of arthroplasty infections belong to the normal skin flora, it is hardly possible to discern between infectious strains and contaminants using swab material. In summary, tissue swabs cannot be recommended to assess prosthetic infections reliably.

3.2.2 Joint aspiration fluid
The overall significance of culture from pre-operative synovial fluid to detect periprosthetic infection is valued as high. However, sensitivity may be reduced if the infection does not involve the synovia or if the concentration of planktonic bacteria in the fluid is limited due to a mature biofilm. Furthermore, false positive results from skin flora occur (Barrack & Harris, 1993; Della Valle et al., 2007; Eisler et al., 2001; Fink et al., 2008; Lachiewicz et al., 1996; Malhotra & Morgan, 2004; Williams et al., 2004).

3.2.3 Periprosthetic tissue biopsies
Analysis of tissue biopsies offers the advantage that multiple samples can be obtained from different locations within the suspicious area. Repeated isolation of bacteria (e. g., isolation of the same organism in at least 2 tissue samples) increases the probability of infection. Thus, there are several reports in which higher sensitivity of tissue culture compared with synovial fluid culture is observed (Fink et al., 2008; Meermans & Haddad, 2010; Roberts et al., 1992; Sadiq et al., 2005; Williams et al., 2004).

3.3 Logistics between clinic and laboratory
Pre-analytical sampling errors have been claimed to contribute significantly to false-negative culture results, with highly sensitive PCR techniques being a means to overcome these drawbacks (Achermann et al., 2010). Guidelines devised by the German Society of Hygiene and Microbiology have proposed that periprosthetic sample material intended for microbiological cultivation should be processed within one hour post-drawing. Although such stringent demands are not realistic for the routine setting, it is indeed crucial to establish a standardized work flow between the clinic and the laboratory regarding the procedures of sample drawing, transportation to the laboratory, and specimen processing. The organizational structure in our laboratory comprises a courier service as well as evening and weekend laboratory duty, which ensures that over 95% of culture samples are processed within 6 hours post-operatively (see 4.1.1).

3.4 Sample processing
The efforts made to obtain significant sample material are futile if the laboratory process is not optimized. However, costs and benefits should be well-balanced.

3.4.1 Native material
The simplest way of tissue sample processing is mincing by a scalpel. This allows efficient investigation of multiple samples from each patient (see 3.2.3). If carried out under a laminar air flow workbench it is not highly prone to contamination (Atkins et al., 1998; Schäfer et al., 2008; Trampuz et al., 2006, 2007).
Some authors favor scraping the surface of the explanted material. This has been reported to be more sensitive than tissue culture but also liable to contamination (Bjerkan et al., 2009; Neut et al., 2003).

3.4.2 Blood culture vials
Automated incubation and fluorometric detection of bacterial growth improves sensitivity compared with conventional liquid culture broths (Font-Vizcarra et al., 2010; Levine & Evans, 2001). However, there are potential drawbacks. Firstly, the possibility to determine leukocyte counts is lost if no native material is saved. Secondly, if the sample volume falls short of three milliliters, standard aerobic and anaerobic blood culture bottles may lack sensitivity. Pediatric vials are optimized for culture of lower sample volumes, but it is possible that some anaerobic bacteria are missed due to the composition of the medium (Morello et al., 1991).

3.4.3 Sonication of explants
Sonication of explanted prosthesis components to disrupt bacterial biofilms has been assessed by several authors (Achermann et al., 2010; Kobayashi et al., 2006; Trampuz et al., 2003, 2007; Tunney et al., 1998). Culture of the sonication fluid appears to be more sensitive than native sample processing. However, it is cumbersome and not suitable for high-throughput analysis. The possible destruction of planktonic bacteria is an issue that has not been raised systematically to date, but may be of importance in cases of prosthetic infection caused by bacteria which do not establish classical biofilms (Sampedro et al., 2010). There also may be an increased risk of contamination (Holinka et al., 2011; Trampuz et al., 2006).

3.4.4 Bead mill processing of tissue biopsies
The bacterial yield using a bead mill is probably enhanced due to facilitated tissue disruption (Roux et al., 2011). However, careful evaluation of conditions for different bacterial species is necessary in order to avoid overheating of samples and mechanical disruption of planktonic bacteria. At present it cannot be decided whether bead mill processing offers significant advantages.

3.5 Identification of infectious agents
3.5.1 Conventional microbiological detection
Direct gram staining of periprosthetic samples is insensitive and therefore not recommended as a routine test (Banit et al., 2002; Parvizi et al., 2006; Spangehl et al., 1999). However, it can be useful in certain cases of early infection, where prompt treatment of agents which show characteristic morphology (e. g. *Clostridium perfringens*) is enabled.
Classic microbiologic culture confirms the presence of viable bacteria and permits testing for antibiotic susceptibility.

3.5.2 PCR strategies
Universal bacterial detection by PCR-based amplification of the 16S rRNA gene allows the identification of bacteria or fungi which are not viable by conventional culture methods. The overall sensitivity may be higher compared with culture (Bergin et al., 2010; Dempsey et al., 2007; Ince et al., 2004; Levine et al., 1995; Panousis et al., 2005; Tunney et al., 1999). On the other hand, singular specific PCR assays (Kobayashi et al., 2009; Piper et al., 2009; Tarkin et al., 2003) or multiplex assays (Achermann et al., 2010) are sensitive but limited to the organisms included in the test panel.

Although important antibiotic resistance mechanisms like methicillin resistance can be identified genotypically with PCR (Kobayashi et al., 2009; Tarkin et al., 2003), for most substance classes phenotypic susceptibility testing will be necessary in the foreseeable future.
There is no straightforward method to determine whether microbial DNA as detected by PCR reflects living organisms. On the other hand, it cannot be ruled out that previous therapy with antibiotics hampers the sensitivity not only of culture, but also of PCR (Achermann et al., 2010).

3.6 Culture conditions
3.6.1 Culture media
A combination of solid (usually blood agar, chocolate agar, and Schaedler agar) and liquid media (e. g. brain-heart infusion broth and Schaedler broth) is used by standard for aerobic and anaerobic cultivation. Solid media alone lack sensitivity to detect low-grade infections because because the medium eventually dries out. On the other hand, infections involving more than one agent can be overlooked if only broth media are utilized because slower-growing organisms may be inhibited in the presence of fast-growing bacteria.

3.6.2 Culture duration
"Standard" cultivation periods (mostly ≤ 7 days in the literature) are generally questionable in infections where biofilms are involved, due to low cell counts of planktonic bacteria and impaired growth rates of sessile organisms in the biofilm. However, the issue was not addressed for a long time. Prolonged cultivation for 14 days was described sporadically (Ince et al., 2004) and even included as a standard recommendation into German practice guidelines, but not assessed under controlled conditions. Thus, our group systematically evaluated a 14-day culture period with periprosthetic tissue samples from hip and knee patients (Schäfer et al., 2008).
Using the algorithm described under 3.1.1 to distinguish infecting agents from contaminating strains, only 74% of the infections (caused by "early" agents) were found within the first week of cultivation (Schäfer et al., 2008). In the second week we not only identified a significant amount of additional infections, but also a completely different spectrum of causative ("late") species (Table 1).

	isolated organisms	frequency (%)	median time to detection (days)
early species	*Staphylococcus aureus*	8.9	2
	coagulase-negative staphylococci	55.4	4
	Enterococcus species	3.8	2
	Streptococcus species	3.8	1.5
	Enterobacteriaceae	1.9	5
late species	coryneform bacteria	7.6	10
	Propionibacterium species	13.4	11
	Finegoldia species	3.2	8
	others	1.9	9.5

Table 1. Spectrum of bacteria detected over a 14-day cultivation period.

Regarding the late species, the sensitivity would have been merely 27% if cultures had been monitored for only 7 days (Fig. 1).

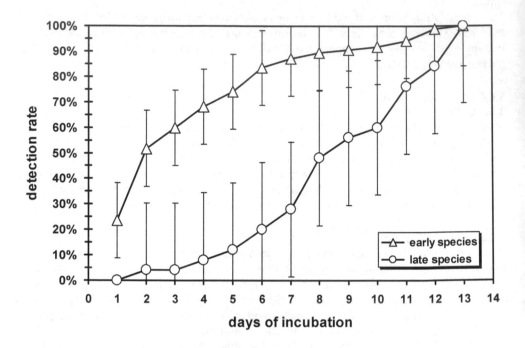

Fig. 1. Detection rates of early and late species depending on the cultivation period. Whisker bars span the Hall-Wellner 95% confidence intervals.

3.7 Discrimination between infection and contamination

There is no standardized procedure which would define infection over contamination accurately. Regarding tissue samples, usually a combined algorithm of neutrophil infiltration scores (2.3.2) and culture detection of identical organisms from multiple tissue samples is used. However, due to the missing consensus criteria the approaches vary considerably between studies (Atkins et al., 1998; Bori et al., 2007; Fink et al., 2008; Ko et al., 2005; Mirra et al., 1976; Pandey et al., 1999).

A problem we encountered was that the algorithms we have adopted to define infections (Atkins et al., 1998; Pandey et al., 1999; Virolainen et al., 2002) were evaluated in the context of "standard" microbiological cultivation periods. Thus, with prolonged culture duration (3.6.2) a larger amount of contaminants might have impaired the significance of this algorithm. However, our findings allowed us to refute the concern that prolonged culture of tissue biopsies could lead to over-proportional contamination rates (Schäfer et al., 2008). It became clear that among both the "early" and the "late" agents (Table 1) a highly significant correlation existed between positive histology and the number of culture-positive tissues (Fig. 2).

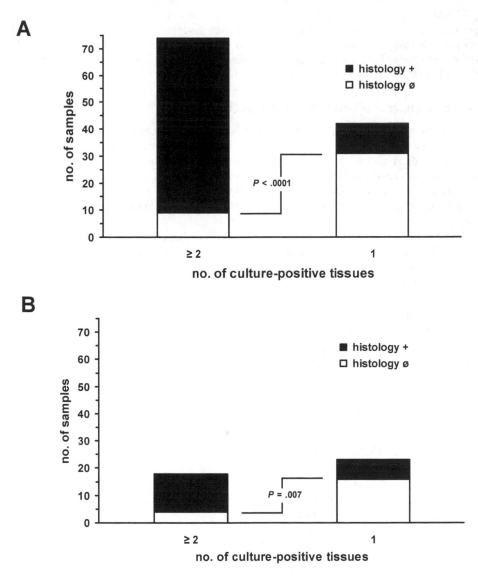

Fig. 2. Correlation between positive histology and the number of culture-positive tissue biopsies. (A) early species. (B) late species. Statistical significance was demonstrated by the χ^2 test.

3.8 Stage at which samples are attained

Although an additional risk and cost factor at first glance, preoperative evaluation of tissue samples in addition to joint aspiration can be helpful to identify the causative agent of arthroplasty infection accurately before the revision is carried out (Fink et al., 2008). This enables a one-stage replacement procedure, if clinically viable. Moreover, it allows to design an individual regimen of systemic and localized antibiotic treatment for two-stage approaches using cement spacers supplemented with antibiotics (Fink et al., 2011). However, the utility of pre-operative biopsies is controversial between studies, mainly due to differences regarding the number of biopsies obtained and the definitions of infection (Fink et al., 2008, 2009; Meermans & Haddad, 2010).

4. Our own approach and future prospects

4.1 The value of both pre-operative and intra-operative sampling

We are convinced that pre-operative identification of the causative agent is a key factor for successful eradication of arthroplasty infections. It enables the design of individualized systemic and localized antibiotic therapy, while intra-operative tissue samples confirm the diagnosis and allow modification of the systemic antibiotic regimen if necessary. The diagnostic workflows we have established to identify hip and knee infections are outlined below.

To minimize the effect of false-negative results, we call for an antibiotic-free interval of 4 weeks before sampling for microbiological diagnosis. At our clinic we withhold peri-operative antibiotic prophylaxis until samples have been drawn, and we have not experienced adverse outcomes.

4.1.1 Samples and diagnosis

An overview of the laboratory procedures is given in Table 2.

sample material	storage	detection method	processing method	no. of samples	definition of infection
synovial aspiration fluid	room temp.	14-day automated culture	pediatric blood culture vial		
tissue biopsies	4°C	14-day aerobic and anaerobic culture sheep blood agar chocolate agar Schaedler agar brain-heart infusion broth Schaedler broth	native	5	identical organisms in ≥ 2 samples
	-20°C	histological staining	frozen sections	5	≥ 5 neutrophils per 400 x field in 10 fields

Table 2. Overview over the laboratory methods used to detect arthroplasty infection.

The definitive diagnosis of arthroplasty infection is established with multiple tissue biopsies taken from the periprosthetic membrane and other macroscopically conspicuous sites during revision surgery. We have experienced that the inflammation process can be assessed with high reliability if 5 samples each are obtained for culture and for histologic analysis. The definition that i) growth of indistinguishable bacteria in ≥ 2 specimens or ii) microbial growth in one specimen combined with a histology score of 3+ (≥ 5 neutrophils per high-power field in 10 fields) (Atkins et al., 1998; Pandey et al., 1999; Virolainen et al., 2002) has proven feasible with respect to the clinical outcomes (Fink et al., 2008, 2009).

Until now we use native tissue biopsies for culture. Tissue mincing is simple to perform and not too prone to contamination if carried out under a laminar air flow workbench. In our opinion, the prolonged incubation period of 14 days we carry out before cultures are cleared is a decisive measure. The persuasiveness of this approach has been shown in detail in 3.6.2. Although it would be interesting to compare the allegedly most sensitive sonication culture method directly with prolonged tissue cultivation, we doubt that the cumbersome and potentially contamination-prone sonication concept would prove significantly superior to our own approach.

As we are convinced that prolonged cultivation over 14 days is the key to detecting infecting organisms with optimal sensitivity, we also currently refrain from using PCR techniques on a routine basis.

If overnight storage of unprocessed samples is necessary, which occurs in less than 5% of cases in our setting, tissue specimens are kept at 4°C and processed at the laboratory the next morning with highly reproducible results. Synovial fluid, when inoculated into pediatric blood culture vials immediately post-drawing, is stable for at least 24 hours at room temperature. Subsequent supplementation with the appropriate enhancing medium, which is necessary to cultivate blood-free sample fluids, can then be done at the laboratory.

Taken together, our diagnostic measures have contributed significantly to the high eradication rates we observe with the treatment of both hip and knee arthroplasty infections (Fink et al., 2008, 2009).

4.1.2 Hip infections

By default, we carry out two-stage revisions of infected hips in our clinic (Fink et al., 2009). Localized antibiotics applied via cement spacer and systemic antibiotics are customized for administration at the time of revision surgery (Fink et al., 2011).

The general sampling algorithm is depicted schematically in Fig. 3. In addition, we obtain pre-operative tissue biopsies for culture and histology if the joint aspiration culture is negative but the risk assessment suggests indicates septic implant failure.

4.1.3 Knee infections

We perform pre-operative tissue biopsies rather than joint aspiration if it is clear that revision operation is necessary due to an unstable implant (Fig. 4). Five biopsies for culture are obtained in a blind fashion without instillating fluid in the intra-articular space (to avoid possible losses in sensitivity due to sample dilution). Afterwards standard arthroscopy is performed to rule out possible joint damage, and during this process 5 additional tissue samples are obtained for histological analysis.

We define infection using the same combined culture and histology algorithm as in biopsy samples taken during revision surgery. Our experience is that pre-operative biopsies are more sensitive than culture from aspirated synovial fluid (Fink et al., 2008).

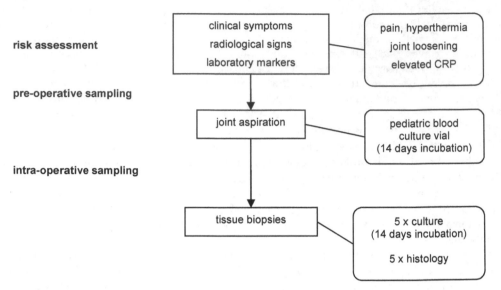

Fig. 3. Sampling algorithm for suspected periprosthetic hip infection. If joint aspiration cultures are negative but the risk assessment suggests indicates septic implant failure, pre-operative tissue biopsies are drawn additionally for culture and histology.

In stable implants, we do not undertake the risk of causing joint damage by blinded tissue biopsy. Instead, joint aspiration culture is performed, which has shown accuracy of 89% (Fink et al., 2008).

The pre-operative diagnostic approach of combined tissue culture histology has shown an accuracy of 98.6% compared to the definitive results obtained during revision surgery (Fink et al., 2008).

4.2 Future prospects

The detection of bacterial RNA rather than DNA by reverse transcription PCR is a potentially useful new approach to arthroplasty infection (Bergin et al., 2010). On one hand, RNA should be present only in viable bacteria and therefore indicate infections more accurately than DNA. On the other hand, the much shorter half-life of RNA should make its presence as a contaminant less likely. It remains to be seen whether this concept will prevail.

Rapid identification of bacteria and fungi to the species level by matrix-assisted laser desorption/ionization time-of-flight (MALDI-TOF) mass spectrometry is utilized increasingly. There are already promising data on the detection of *Staphylococcus epidermidis* in tissue samples of patients with periprosthetic joint infections (Harris et al., 2010). It appears that it should even be possible in the near future to prove clonal identity of strains from the same species isolated from different tissue samples with this technique. This should facilitate the decision whether bacteria isolated from multiple tissue biopsies are likely to be involved in infection or rather reflect contaminating strains.

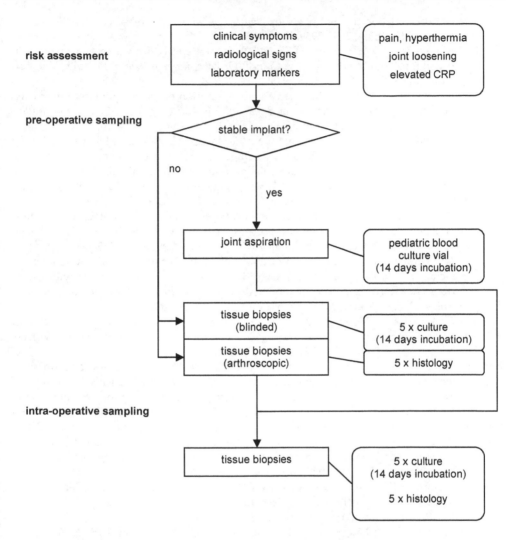

Fig. 4. Sampling algorithm for suspected periprosthetic knee infection.

5. References

Achermann, Y.; Vogt, M.; Leunig, M.; Wust, J. & Trampuz, A. (2010). Improved diagnosis of periprosthetic joint infection by multiplex PCR of sonication fluid from removed implants. *Journal of Clinical Microbiology*, Vol. 48, No. 4, (April 2010), pp. 1208-1214, ISSN 1098-660X

Atkins, B.L.; Athanasou, N.; Deeks, J.J.; Crook, D.W.; Simpson, H.; Peto, T.E.; McLardy-Smith, P. & Berendt, A.R. (1998). Prospective evaluation of criteria for microbiological diagnosis of prosthetic-joint infection at revision arthroplasty. The

OSIRIS Collaborative Study Group. *Journal of Clinical Microbiology*, Vol. 36, No. 10, (October 1998), pp. 2932-2939, ISSN 0095-1137

Banit, D.M.; Kaufer, H. & Hartford, J.M. (2002). Intraoperative frozen section analysis in revision total joint arthroplasty. *Clinical Orthopaedics and Related Research*, Vol. 401, (August 2002), pp. 230-238, ISSN 0009-921X

Barrack, R.L. & Harris, W.H. (1993). The value of aspiration of the hip joint before revision total hip arthroplasty. *Journal of Bone and Joint Surgery*, Vol. 75, No. 1, (January 1993), pp. 66-76, ISSN 0021-9355

Bejon, P.; Berendt, A.; Atkins, B.L.; Green, N.; Parry, H.; Masters, S.; McLardy-Smith, P.; Gundle, R. & Byren, I. (2010). Two-stage revision for prosthetic joint infection: predictors of outcome and the role of reimplantation microbiology. *Journal of Antimicrobial Chemotherapy*, Vol. 65, No. 3, (Mar 2010), pp. 569-575, ISSN 1460-2091

Berbari, E.; Mabry, T.; Tsaras, G.; Spangehl, M.; Erwin, P.J.; Murad, M.H.; Steckelberg, J. & Osmon, D. (2010). Inflammatory blood laboratory levels as markers of prosthetic joint infection: a systematic review and meta-analysis. *Journal of Bone and Joint Surgery*, Vol. 92, No. 11, (September 2010), pp. 2102-2109, ISSN 1535-1386

Bergin, P.F.; Doppelt, J.D.; Hamilton, W.G.; Mirick, G.E.; Jones, A.E.; Sritulanondha, S.; Helm, J.M. & Tuan, R.S. (2010). Detection of periprosthetic infections with use of ribosomal RNA-based polymerase chain reaction. *Journal of Bone and Joint Surgery*, Vol. 92, No. 3, (March 2010), pp. 654-663, ISSN 1535-1386

Bjerkan, G.; Witso, E. & Bergh, K. (2009). Sonication is superior to scraping for retrieval of bacteria in biofilm on titanium and steel surfaces in vitro. *Acta Orthopaedica*, Vol. 80, No. 2, (April 2009), pp. 245-250, ISSN 1745-3682

Bori, G.; Soriano, A.; Garcia, S.; Mallofre, C.; Riba, J. & Mensa, J. (2007). Usefulness of histological analysis for predicting the presence of microorganisms at the time of reimplantation after hip resection arthroplasty for the treatment of infection. *Journal of Bone and Joint Surgery*, Vol. 89, No. 6, (June 2007), pp. 1232-1237, ISSN 0021-9355

Bottner, F.; Wegner, A.; Winkelmann, W.; Becker, K.; Erren, M. & Götze, C. (2007). Interleukin-6, procalcitonin and TNF-alpha: markers of periprosthetic infection following total joint replacement. *Journal of Bone and Joint Surgery. British Volume*, Vol. 89, No. 1, (January 2007), pp. 94-99, ISSN 0301-620X

Bozic, K.J.; Kurtz, S.M.; Lau, E.; Ong, K.; Vail, T.P. & Berry, D.J. (2009). The epidemiology of revision total hip arthroplasty in the United States. *Journal of Bone and Joint Surgery*, Vol. 91, No. 1, (January 2009), pp. 128-133, ISSN 1535-1386

Bozic, K.J.; Kurtz, S.M.; Lau, E.; Ong, K.; Chiu, V.; Vail, T.P.; Rubash, H.E. & Berry, D.J. (2010). The epidemiology of revision total knee arthroplasty in the United States. *Clinical Orthopaedics and Related Research*, Vol. 468, No. 1, (January 2010), pp. 45-51, ISSN 0009-921X

Costerton, J.W.; Stewart, P.S. & Greenberg, E.P. (1999). Bacterial biofilms: a common cause of persistent infections. *Science*, Vol. 284, No. 5418, (May 1999), pp. 1318-1322, ISSN 0036-8075

Cui, Q.; Mihalko, W.M.; Shields, J.S.; Ries, M. & Saleh, K.J. (2007). Antibiotic-impregnated cement spacers for the treatment of infection associated with total hip or knee arthroplasty. *Journal of Bone and Joint Surgery*, Vol. 89, No. 4, (April 2007), pp. 871-882, ISSN 0021-9355

Cune, J.; Soriano, A.; Martinez, J.C.; Garcia, S. & Mensa, J. (2009). A superficial swab culture is useful for microbiologic diagnosis in acute prosthetic joint infections. *Clinical Orthopaedics and Related Research*, Vol. 467, No. 2, (February 2009), pp. 531-535, ISSN 0009-921X

Della Valle, C.; Parvizi, J.; Bauer, T.W.; Dicesare, P.E.; Evans, R.P.; Segreti, J.; Spangehl, M.; Watters, W.C., 3rd; Keith, M.; Turkelson, C.M.; Wies, J.L.; Sluka, P. & Hitchcock, K. (2010). Diagnosis of periprosthetic joint infections of the hip and knee. *Journal of the American Academy of Orthopaedic Surgeons*, Vol. 18, No. 12, (December 2010), pp. 760-770, ISSN 1067-151X

Della Valle, C.J.; Sporer, S.M.; Jacobs, J.J.; Berger, R.A.; Rosenberg, A.G. & Paprosky, W.G. (2007). Preoperative testing for sepsis before revision total knee arthroplasty. *Journal of Arthroplasty*, Vol. 22, No. 6 Suppl 2, (September 2007), pp. 90-93, ISSN 0883-5403

Dempsey, K.E.; Riggio, M.P.; Lennon, A.; Hannah, V.E.; Ramage, G.; Allan, D. & Bagg, J. (2007). Identification of bacteria on the surface of clinically infected and non-infected prosthetic hip joints removed during revision arthroplasties by 16S rRNA gene sequencing and by microbiological culture. *Arthritis Res Ther*, Vol. 9, No. 3, (May 2007), pp. R46, ISSN 1478-6362

Di Cesare, P.E.; Chang, E.; Preston, C.F. & Liu, C.J. (2005). Serum interleukin-6 as a marker of periprosthetic infection following total hip and knee arthroplasty. *Journal of Bone and Joint Surgery*, Vol. 87, No. 9, (Sep 2005), pp. 1921-1927, ISSN 0021-9355

Donlan, R.M. & Costerton, J.W. (2002). Biofilms: survival mechanisms of clinically relevant microorganisms. *Clinical Microbiology Reviews*, Vol. 15, No. 2, (April 2002), pp. 167-193, ISSN 0893-8512

Donlan, R.M. (2005). New approaches for the characterization of prosthetic joint biofilms. *Clinical Orthopaedics and Related Research*, Vol. 437, (August 2005), pp. 12-19, ISSN 0009-921X

Eisler, T.; Svensson, O.; Engström, C.F.; Reinholt, F.P.; Lundberg, C.; Wejkner, B.; Schmalholz, A. & Elmstedt, E. (2001). Ultrasound for diagnosis of infection in revision total hip arthroplasty. *Journal of Arthroplasty*, Vol. 16, No. 8, (December 2001), pp. 1010-1017, ISSN 0883-5403

Engesaeter, L.B.; Lie, S.A.; Espehaug, B.; Furnes, O.; Vollset, S.E. & Havelin, L.I. (2003). Antibiotic prophylaxis in total hip arthroplasty: effects of antibiotic prophylaxis systemically and in bone cement on the revision rate of 22,170 primary hip replacements followed 0-14 years in the Norwegian Arthroplasty Register. *Acta Orthopaedica Scandinavica*, Vol. 74, No. 6, (December 2003), pp. 644-651, ISSN 0001-6470

Fehring, T.K. & McAlister, J.A., Jr. (1994). Frozen histologic section as a guide to sepsis in revision joint arthroplasty. *Clinical Orthopaedics and Related Research*, Vol. 304, (July 1994), pp. 229-237, ISSN 0009-921X

Fink, B.; Makowiak, C.; Fuerst, M.; Berger, I.; Schäfer, P. & Frommelt, L. (2008). The value of synovial biopsy, joint aspiration and C-reactive protein in the diagnosis of late periprosthetic infection of total knee replacements. *Journal of Bone and Joint Surgery. British Volume*, Vol. 90, No. 7, (July 2008), pp. 874-878, ISSN 0301-620X

Fink, B.; Grossmann, A.; Fuerst, M.; Schäfer, P. & Frommelt, L. (2009). Two-stage cementless revision of infected hip endoprostheses. *Clinical Orthopaedics and Related Research,* Vol. 467, No. 7, (July 2009), pp. 1848-1858, ISSN 0009-921X

Fink, B.; Vogt, S.; Reinsch, M. & Buchner, H. (2011). Sufficient Release of Antibiotic by a Spacer 6 Weeks after Implantation in Two-stage Revision of Infected Hip Prostheses. *Clinical Orthopaedics and Related Research,* in press

Font-Vizcarra, L.; Garcia, S.; Martinez-Pastor, J.C.; Sierra, J.M. & Soriano, A. (2010). Blood culture flasks for culturing synovial fluid in prosthetic joint infections. *Clinical Orthopaedics and Related Research,* Vol. 468, No. 8, (August 2010), pp. 2238-2243, ISSN 0009-921X

Frances Borrego, A.; Martinez, F.M.; Cebrian Parra, J.L.; Graneda, D.S.; Crespo, R.G. & Lopez-Duran Stern, L. (2007). Diagnosis of infection in hip and knee revision surgery: intraoperative frozen section analysis. *International Orthopaedics,* Vol. 31, No. 1, (February 2007), pp. 33-37, ISSN 0341-2695

Ghanem, E.; Parvizi, J.; Burnett, R.S.; Sharkey, P.F.; Keshavarzi, N.; Aggarwal, A. & Barrack, R.L. (2008). Cell count and differential of aspirated fluid in the diagnosis of infection at the site of total knee arthroplasty. *Journal of Bone and Joint Surgery,* Vol. 90, No. 8, (August 2008), pp. 1637-1643, ISSN 1535-1386

Gomez, E. & Patel, R. (2011a). Laboratory diagnosis of prosthetic joint infection, Part I. *Clinical Microbiology Newsletter,* Vol. 33, No. 8, (April 2011), pp. 55-60, ISSN 0196-4399

Gomez, E. & Patel, R. (2011b). Laboratory diagnosis of prosthetic joint infection, Part II. *Clinical Microbiology Newsletter,* Vol. 33, No. 9, (May 2011), pp. 63-70, ISSN 0196-4399

Greidanus, N.V.; Masri, B.A.; Garbuz, D.S.; Wilson, S.D.; McAlinden, M.G.; Xu, M. & Duncan, C.P. (2007). Use of erythrocyte sedimentation rate and C-reactive protein level to diagnose infection before revision total knee arthroplasty. A prospective evaluation. *Journal of Bone and Joint Surgery,* Vol. 89, No. 7, (July 2007), pp. 1409-1416, ISSN 0021-9355

Gristina, A.G. & Costerton, J.W. (1985). Bacterial adherence to biomaterials and tissue. The significance of its role in clinical sepsis. *Journal of Bone and Joint Surgery,* Vol. 67, No. 2, (February 1985), pp. 264-273, ISSN 0021-9355

Hanssen, A.D. & Osmon, D.R. (2002). Evaluation of a staging system for infected hip arthroplasty. *Clinical Orthopaedics and Related Research,* Vol. 403, (October 2002), pp. 16-22, ISSN 0009-921X

Harris, L.G.; El-Bouri, K.; Johnston, S.; Rees, E.; Frommelt, L.; Siemssen, N.; Christner, M.; Davies, A.P.; Rohde, H. & Mack, D. (2010). Rapid identification of staphylococci from prosthetic joint infections using MALDI-TOF mass-spectrometry. *International Journal of Artificial Organs,* Vol. 33, No. 9, (September 2010), pp. 568-574, ISSN 1724-6040

Holinka, J.; Bauer, L.; Hirschl, A.M.; Graninger, W.; Windhager, R. & Presterl, E. (2011). Sonication cultures of explanted components as an add-on test to routinely conducted microbiological diagnostics improve pathogen detection. *Journal of Orthopaedic Research,* Vol. 29, No. 4, (April 2011), pp. 617-622, ISSN 1554-527X

Ince, A.; Rupp, J.; Frommelt, L.; Katzer, A.; Gille, J. & Löhr, J.F. (2004). Is "aseptic" loosening of the prosthetic cup after total hip replacement due to nonculturable bacterial pathogens in patients with low-grade infection? *Clinical Infectious Diseases*, Vol. 39, No. 11, (December 2004), pp. 1599-1603, ISSN 1537-6591

Jämsen, E.; Huhtala, H.; Puolakka, T. & Moilanen, T. (2009). Risk factors for infection after knee arthroplasty. A register-based analysis of 43,149 cases. *Journal of Bone and Joint Surgery*, Vol. 91, No. 1, (January 2009), pp. 38-47, ISSN 1535-1386

Jones, S.M.; Morgan, M.; Humphrey, T.J. & Lappin-Scott, H. (2001). Effect of vancomycin and rifampicin on meticillin-resistant Staphylococcus aureus biofilms. *Lancet*, Vol. 357, No. 9249, (January 2001), pp. 40-41, ISSN 0140-6736

Kamme, C. & Lindberg, L. (1981). Aerobic and anaerobic bacteria in deep infections after total hip arthroplasty: differential diagnosis between infectious and non-infectious loosening. *Clinical Orthopaedics and Related Research*, Vol. 154, (January-February 1981), pp. 201-207, ISSN 0009-921X

Ko, P.S.; Ip, D.; Chow, K.P.; Cheung, F.; Lee, O.B. & Lam, J.J. (2005). The role of intraoperative frozen section in decision making in revision hip and knee arthroplasties in a local community hospital. *Journal of Arthroplasty*, Vol. 20, No. 2, (February 2005), pp. 189-195, ISSN 0883-5403

Kobayashi, N.; Bauer, T.W.; Sakai, H.; Togawa, D.; Lieberman, I.H.; Fujishiro, T. & Procop, G.W. (2006). The use of newly developed real-time PCR for the rapid identification of bacteria in culture-negative osteomyelitis. *Joint Bone Spine*, Vol. 73, No. 6, (December 2006), pp. 745-747, ISSN 1778-7254

Kobayashi, N.; Inaba, Y.; Choe, H.; Iwamoto, N.; Ishida, T.; Yukizawa, Y.; Aoki, C.; Ike, H. & Saito, T. (2009). Rapid and sensitive detection of methicillin-resistant Staphylococcus periprosthetic infections using real-time polymerase chain reaction. *Diagnostic Microbiology and Infectious Disease*, Vol. 64, No. 2, (June 2009), pp. 172-176, ISSN 1879-0070

Krenn, V.; Morawietz, L.; Jakobs, M.; Kienapfel, H.; Ascherl, R.; Bause, L.; Kuhn, H.; Matziolis, G.; Skutek, M. & Gehrke, T. (2011). Joint endoprosthesis pathology: Histopathological diagnostics and classification. *Pathologe*, Vol. 32, No. 3, (May 2011), pp. 210-219, ISSN 0172-8113

Lachiewicz, P.F.; Rogers, G.D. & Thomason, H.C. (1996). Aspiration of the hip joint before revision total hip arthroplasty. Clinical and laboratory factors influencing attainment of a positive culture. *Journal of Bone and Joint Surgery*, Vol. 78, No. 5, (May 1996), pp. 749-754, ISSN 0021-9355

Levine, B.R. & Evans, B.G. (2001). Use of blood culture vial specimens in intraoperative detection of infection. *Clinical Orthopaedics and Related Research*, Vol. 382, (January 2001), pp. 222-231, ISSN 0009-921X

Levine, M.J.; Mariani, B.A.; Tuan, R.S. & Booth, R.E., Jr. (1995). Molecular genetic diagnosis of infected total joint arthroplasty. *Journal of Arthroplasty*, Vol. 10, No. 1, (February 1995), pp. 93-94, ISSN 0883-5403

Lonner, J.H.; Desai, P.; Dicesare, P.E.; Steiner, G. & Zuckerman, J.D. (1996). The reliability of analysis of intraoperative frozen sections for identifying active infection during revision hip or knee arthroplasty. *Journal of Bone and Joint Surgery*, Vol. 78, No. 10, (October 1996), pp. 1553-1558, ISSN 0021-9355

Malhotra, R. & Morgan, D.A. (2004). Role of core biopsy in diagnosing infection before revision hip arthroplasty. *Journal of Arthroplasty*, Vol. 19, No. 1, (January 2004), pp. 78-87, ISSN 0883-5403

Meermans, G. & Haddad, F.S. (2010). Is there a role for tissue biopsy in the diagnosis of periprosthetic infection? *Clinical Orthopaedics and Related Research*, Vol. 468, No. 5, (May 2010), pp. 1410-1417, ISSN 1528-1132

Mirra, J.M.; Amstutz, H.C.; Matos, M. & Gold, R. (1976). The pathology of the joint tissues and its clinical relevance in prosthesis failure. *Clinical Orthopaedics and Related Research*, Vol. No. 117, (June 1976), pp. 221-240, ISSN 0009-921X

Monzon, M.; Oteiza, C.; Leiva, J.; Lamata, M. & Amorena, B. (2002). Biofilm testing of Staphylococcus epidermidis clinical isolates: low performance of vancomycin in relation to other antibiotics. *Diagnostic Microbiology and Infectious Disease*, Vol. 44, No. 4, (December 2002), pp. 319-324, ISSN 0732-8893

Morawietz, L.; Classen, R.A.; Schröder, J.H.; Dynybil, C.; Perka, C.; Skwara, A.; Neidel, J.; Gehrke, T.; Frommelt, L.; Hansen, T.; Otto, M.; Barden, B.; Aigner, T.; Stiehl, P.; Schubert, T.; Meyer-Scholten, C.; König, A.; Ströbel, P.; Rader, C.P.; Kirschner, S.; Lintner, F.; Rüther, W.; Bos, I.; Hendrich, C.; Kriegsmann, J. & Krenn, V. (2006). Proposal for a histopathological consensus classification of the periprosthetic interface membrane. *Journal of Clinical Pathology*, Vol. 59, No. 6, (June 2006), pp. 591-597, ISSN 0021-9746

Morello, J.A.; Matushek, S.M.; Dunne, W.M. & Hinds, D.B. (1991). Performance of a BACTEC nonradiometric medium for pediatric blood cultures. *Journal of Clinical Microbiology*, Vol. 29, No. 2, (February 1991), pp. 359-362, ISSN 0095-1137

Neut, D.; Van Horn, J.R.; Van Kooten, T.G.; Van Der Mei, H.C. & Busscher, H.J. (2003). Detection of biomaterial-associated infections in orthopaedic joint implants. *Clinical Orthopaedics and Related Research*, Vol. No. 413, (August 2003), pp. 261-268, ISSN 0009-921X

Nunez, L.V.; Buttaro, M.A.; Morandi, A.; Pusso, R. & Piccaluga, F. (2007). Frozen sections of samples taken intraoperatively for diagnosis of infection in revision hip surgery. *Acta Orthopaedica*, Vol. 78, No. 2, (April 2007), pp. 226-230, ISSN 1745-3674

Pandey, R.; Drakoulakis, E. & Athanasou, N.A. (1999). An assessment of the histological criteria used to diagnose infection in hip revision arthroplasty tissues. *Journal of Clinical Pathology*, Vol. 52, No. 2, (February 1999), pp. 118-123, ISSN 0021-9746

Panousis, K.; Grigoris, P.; Butcher, I.; Rana, B.; Reilly, J.H. & Hamblen, D.L. (2005). Poor predictive value of broad-range PCR for the detection of arthroplasty infection in 92 cases. *Acta Orthopaedica*, Vol. 76, No. 3, (June 2005), pp. 341-346, ISSN 1745-3674

Parvizi, J.; Ghanem, E.; Menashe, S.; Barrack, R.L. & Bauer, T.W. (2006). Periprosthetic infection: what are the diagnostic challenges? *Journal of Bone and Joint Surgery*, Vol. 88 Suppl 4, (December 2006), pp. 138-147, ISSN 0021-9355

Peel, T.N.; Buising, K.L. & Choong, P.F. (2011). Prosthetic joint infection: challenges of diagnosis and treatment. *ANZ Journal of Surgery*, Vol. 81, No. 1-2, (January 2011), pp. 32-39, ISSN 1445-2197

Piper, K.E.; Jacobson, M.J.; Cofield, R.H.; Sperling, J.W.; Sanchez-Sotelo, J.; Osmon, D.R.; Mcdowell, A.; Patrick, S.; Steckelberg, J.M.; Mandrekar, J.N.; Fernandez Sampedro, M. & Patel, R. (2009). Microbiologic diagnosis of prosthetic shoulder infection by use of implant sonication. *Journal of Clinical Microbiology*, Vol. 47, No. 6, (June 2009), pp. 1878-1884, ISSN 1098-660X

Roberts, P.; Walters, A.J. & Mcminn, D.J. (1992). Diagnosing infection in hip replacements. The use of fine-needle aspiration and radiometric culture. *Journal of Bone and Joint Surgery. British Volume*, Vol. 74, No. 2, (March 1992), pp. 265-269, ISSN 0301-620X

Roux, A.L.; Sivadon-Tardy, V.; Bauer, T.; Lortat-Jacob, A.; Herrmann, J.L.; Gaillard, J.L. & Rottman, M. (2011). Diagnosis of prosthetic joint infection by beadmill processing of a periprosthetic specimen. *Clinical Microbiology and Infection*, Vol. 17, No. 3, (March 2011), pp. 447-450, ISSN 1469-0691

Sadiq, S.; Wootton, J.R.; Morris, C.A. & Northmore-Ball, M.D. (2005). Application of core biopsy in revision arthroplasty for deep infection. *Journal of Arthroplasty*, Vol. 20, No. 2, (February 2005), pp. 196-201, ISSN 0883-5403

Sampedro, M.F.; Huddleston, P.M.; Piper, K.E.; Karau, M.J.; Dekutoski, M.B.; Yaszemski, M.J.; Currier, B.L.; Mandrekar, J.N.; Osmon, D.R.; Mcdowell, A.; Patrick, S.; Steckelberg, J.M. & Patel, R. (2010). A biofilm approach to detect bacteria on removed spinal implants. *Spine*, Vol. 35, No. 12, (May 2010), pp. 1218-1224, ISSN 1528-1159

Schäfer, P.; Fink, B.; Sandow, D.; Margull, A.; Berger, I. & Frommelt, L. (2008). Prolonged bacterial culture to identify late periprosthetic joint infection: a promising strategy. *Clinical Infectious Diseases*, Vol. 47, No. 11, (December 2008), pp. 1403-1409, ISSN 1058-4838

Schinsky, M.F.; Della Valle, C.J.; Sporer, S.M. & Paprosky, W.G. (2008). Perioperative testing for joint infection in patients undergoing revision total hip arthroplasty. *Journal of Bone and Joint Surgery*, Vol. 90, No. 9, (September 2008), pp. 1869-1875, ISSN 1535-1386

Spangehl, M.J.; Masterson, E.; Masri, B.A.; O'connell, J.X. & Duncan, C.P. (1999). The role of intraoperative gram stain in the diagnosis of infection during revision total hip arthroplasty. *Journal of Arthroplasty*, Vol. 14, No. 8, (December 1999), pp. 952-956, ISSN 0883-5403

Stewart, P.S. & Costerton, J.W. (2001). Antibiotic resistance of bacteria in biofilms. *Lancet*, Vol. 358, No. 9276, (July 2001), pp. 135-138, ISSN 0140-6736

Tarkin, I.S.; Henry, T.J.; Fey, P.I.; Iwen, P.C.; Hinrichs, S.H. & Garvin, K.L. (2003). PCR rapidly detects methicillin-resistant staphylococci periprosthetic infection. *Clinical Orthopaedics and Related Research*, Vol. No. 414, (September 2003), pp. 89-94, ISSN 0009-921X

Trampuz, A.; Osmon, D.R.; Hanssen, A.D.; Steckelberg, J.M. & Patel, R. (2003). Molecular and antibiofilm approaches to prosthetic joint infection. *Clinical Orthopaedics and Related Research*, Vol. No. 414, (September 2003), pp. 69-88, ISSN 0009-921X

Trampuz, A.; Hanssen, A.D.; Osmon, D.R.; Mandrekar, J.; Steckelberg, J.M. & Patel, R. (2004). Synovial fluid leukocyte count and differential for the diagnosis of prosthetic knee infection. *American Journal of Medicine*, Vol. 117, No. 8, (October 2004), pp. 556-562, ISSN 0002-9343

Trampuz, A.; Piper, K.E.; Hanssen, A.D.; Osmon, D.R.; Cockerill, F.R.; Steckelberg, J.M. & Patel, R. (2006). Sonication of explanted prosthetic components in bags for diagnosis of prosthetic joint infection is associated with risk of contamination. *Journal of Clinical Microbiology*, Vol. 44, No. 2, (February 2006), pp. 628-631, ISSN 0095-1137

Trampuz, A.; Piper, K.E.; Jacobson, M.J.; Hanssen, A.D.; Unni, K.K.; Osmon, D.R.; Mandrekar, J.N.; Cockerill, F.R.; Steckelberg, J.M.; Greenleaf, J.F. & Patel, R. (2007). Sonication of removed hip and knee prostheses for diagnosis of infection. *New England Journal of Medicine*, Vol. 357, No. 7, (August 2007), pp. 654-663, ISSN 1533-4406

Tunney, M.M.; Patrick, S.; Gorman, S.P.; Nixon, J.R.; Anderson, N.; Davis, R.I.; Hanna, D. & Ramage, G. (1998). Improved detection of infection in hip replacements. A currently underestimated problem. *Journal of Bone and Joint Surgery. British Volume*, Vol. 80, No. 4, (July 1998), pp. 568-572, ISSN 0301-620X

Tunney, M.M.; Patrick, S.; Curran, M.D.; Ramage, G.; Hanna, D.; Nixon, J.R.; Gorman, S.P.; Davis, R.I. & Anderson, N. (1999). Detection of prosthetic hip infection at revision arthroplasty by immunofluorescence microscopy and PCR amplification of the bacterial 16S rRNA gene. *Journal of Clinical Microbiology*, Vol. 37, No. 10, (October 1999), pp. 3281-3290, ISSN 0095-1137

Virolainen, P.; Lähteenmäki, H.; Hiltunen, A.; Sipola, E.; Meurman, O. & Nelimarkka, O. (2002). The reliability of diagnosis of infection during revision arthroplasties. *Scandinavian Journal of Surgery*, Vol. 91, No. 2, (August 2002), pp. 178-181, ISSN 1457-4969

Williams, J.L.; Norman, P. & Stockley, I. (2004). The value of hip aspiration versus tissue biopsy in diagnosing infection before exchange hip arthroplasty surgery. *Journal of Arthroplasty*, Vol. 19, No. 5, (August 2004), pp. 582-586, ISSN 0883-5403

Zimmerli, W.; Trampuz, A. & Ochsner, P.E. (2004). Prosthetic-joint infections. *New England Journal of Medicine*, Vol. 351, No. 16, (October 2004), pp. 1645-1654, ISSN 1533-4406

2

Infection in Primary Hip and Knee Arthroplasty

Michelle M. Dowsey, Trisha N. Peel and Peter F.M. Choong
University of Melbourne, Department of Surgery, St. Vincent's Hospital Melbourne
Department of Orthopaedics, St. Vincent's Hospital Melbourne
Australia

1. Introduction

Since the advent of prosthetic joint replacement, patients suffering from bone and joint pathology have benefited from significant improvements in mobility and pain relief. In Australia 39,200 hip replacements and 39,500 knee replacements were performed in 2009 (Australian Orthopaedic Association National Joint Replacement Registry [AOA NJRR]) (Graves, et al. 2010). With an ageing population, the number of patients undergoing these procedures is projected to increase significantly over time. Data from the United States of America predicts that by 2030, the number of patients undergoing primary hip and knee replacement will increase by 174% and 673% respectively (Kurtz, et al. 2007). The major complication of such techniques is infection of the prosthetic device, which is associated with significant costs to individual patients and to the public health system. Significant morbidity is associated with prosthetic joint infections including the need for further operative procedures, long-term antibiotic therapy, and prolonged hospitalisation. Thereafter, the mortality rate from prosthetic joint infection is estimated to be between 1.0 to 2.7 precent (Ahnfelt, et al. 1990, Zimmerli 2006, Zimmerli, et al. 2004). Aside from the effects on the individual patient, the financial cost to the health system is considerable. The estimated hospital costs is $ 96 166 (US) per patient requiring revision arthroplasty for infection, which is 4.8 times the cost of a primary arthroplasty(Bozic & Ries 2005).

This chapter examines the underlying epidemiology, diagnosis, treatment and challenges in managing this problem.

2. Epidemiology

2.1 Incidence

Identification of prosthetic joint infection currently relies on diagnostic criteria, which include: histopathologic evidence of acute inflammation of periprosthetic tissue, presence of a sinus tract, macroscopic purulence surrounding the prosthesis observed intraoperatively or two or more positive microbiological cultures with the same organism isolated from the prosthetic joint fluid or tissue(Berbari, et al. 1998). We report a rate of prosthetic joint infection between 1.0 – 2.0% in primary lower limb arthroplasty and this is congruent with current literature (Dowsey & Choong 2008, 2009, Swan, et al. 2011). In the United States the rate of infection in knee and hip arthroplasty was 0.92% and 0.88% respectively in a recent review of Medicare data. (Kurtz, et al. 2008). The majority of arthroplasty infections occur in the two years following prosthetic joint surgery. The incidence of knee arthroplasty infection within 2 years was 1.55% decreasing to 0.46% in the subsequent 8 years. Corresponding data in the hip arthroplasty population showed an incidence of 1.63% within 2 years and 0.59% between two to ten years (Kurtz, et al. 2010, Ong, et al. 2009)

2.2 Risk factors

A number of preoperative risk factors for prosthetic joint infection have been identified and these include pre-existing patient co-morbidities such as obesity, diabetes mellitus, rheumatoid arthritis and a history of prior malignancy. Body mass index (BMI) greater than $40kg/m^2$ has been associated with a 9 fold increased risk of knee infection in our series (Dowsey & Choong 2009). Similar studies have shown that for every 1 kg/m^2 increase in body mass index, there was an associated 8% increase in the risk of deep prosthetic joint infection. The association between obesity and deep prosthetic infections is particularly marked in the hip arthroplasty population with the risk of infection increasing from 0.9% in patients within the normal weight range, to 9.1% in morbidly obese(Choong, et al. 2007, Dowsey & Choong 2008). Diabetes mellitus also predisposes patients to deep prosthetic joint infection with 5.3% of diabetic patients developing a prosthetic joint infection in one study (Dowsey & Choong 2009, Yang, et al. 2001). Postulated mechanisms for the increased risk include impaired leucocyte function and impaired wound healing in diabetic patients. Rheumatoid arthritis has been associated with a higher risk of deep prosthetic joint infections. Patients with rheumatoid arthritis have been reported to have a greater than 2.5 fold increase in the risk of arthroplasty infection compared to patients with osteoarthritis (Bengtson & Knutson 1991, Poss, et al. 1984). Whether this is due to impaired immunity secondary to the underlying disease or whether it is a reflection of the increased use of immunosuppressive medications in this cohort remains unclear (Berbari, et al. 2006b). A diagnosis of malignancy not involving the index joint has been identified as a risk factor for the subsequent development of prosthetic joint infection(Berbari, et al. 1998).

Operative risk factors associated with deep prosthetic joint infection include higher American Society of Anaesthesiologist's (ASA) and National Nosocomial Infections Surveillance (NNIS) scores, bilateral surgery, knee arthroplasty, arthroplasty type and operating room conditions. Berbari et al showed that increasing NNIS score was associated with increasing risk of deep prosthetic joint infection; NNIS score 1 was associated with a 1.7 fold increase, increasing to 3.9 with a NNIS score of 2 (Berbari, et al. 1998). The ASA score, a component of the NNIS score, was also associated with an increased risk of arthroplasty infections (Pulido, et al. 2008). Pulido et al identified close to a six-fold increase in risk of prosthetic joint infection in patients undergoing simultaneous bilateral arthroplasty surgery. In the same study, knee arthroplasty, when compared to hip arthroplasty, was independently associated with a higher risk of developing deep prosthetic joint infection (Pulido, et al. 2008). The type of prosthesis used also appears to influence the risk of infection. A 20-fold increased risk of infection with metal hinged prosthetic knee joints compared to metal-to-plastic prostheses has been reported (Poss, et al. 1984).

A number of postoperative risk factors for prosthetic joint infection have also been identified. The most important of these appears to be postoperative wound complications including the presence of superficial infection and/or wound discharge (Bengtson & Knutson 1991, Surin, et al. 1983, Wymenga, et al. 1992). Superficial infection, occurs within 30 days of the operative procedure, only involves the superficial structures and additionally includes one of the following features: purulent discharge, isolation of micro-organisms through aseptic sampling techniques or clinical features of infection (Horan, et al. 1992). Applying this definition, patients with a postoperative surgical site infection had around a 36 fold increase in the risk of the subsequent development of a deep prosthetic wound in one study(Berbari, et al. 1998). Similarly, in another study examining patients with deep prosthetic infections acquired in the perioperative period, 25 of the 26 patients described preceding wound complications, which included; the persistent drainage of fluid from the wound, development of a haematoma under the wound, a superficial infection or a stitch abscesses (Poss, et al. 1984). Of note we have demonstrated that the use of closed suction drainage in total knee arthroplasty is protective of prosthetic knee infection and this may be due the role of a drainage tube in minimizing haematoma formation (Dowsey & Choong 2009). Early post-operative persistent discharge of fluid from the wound has been associated with a 3.2 times higher risk of deep prosthetic joint infection. Often in these cases the same pathogenic organisms isolated from the discharging fluid is later recovered at time of reoperation on the infected hip (Surin, et al. 1983).

Postoperative medical complications including atrial fibrillation and myocardial infarction have also been implicated as risk factors for deep prosthetic joint infection, with a 6-fold and 20-fold respective increase reported (Pulido, et al. 2008). One postulated mechanism to account for this association is that standard management of these medical conditions includes anticoagulation. In the postoperative period this may increase the risk of bleeding and haematoma formation near the wound, which in itself may increase the risk of infection. Secondly, these medical complications may necessitate longer inpatient hospital stay, which may be associated with nosocomial acquisition of infection. Allogenic blood transfusion was also identified as conferring a twofold increased risk of prosthetic infection, again the risk may be via an association with bleeding and haematoma formation near the wound, or possibly as a marker of complications and prolonged hospitalisation (Pulido, et al. 2008).

Nosocomial infections, particularly urinary tract infections have also been identified as risk factors for deep prosthetic joint infections. Surin et al demonstrated that patients with remote infections in the postoperative period were three times more likely to develop deep infections. Over three quarters of these infections were urinary tract infections. Interestingly however, there was no correlation between causative agents of the nosocomial infection and the micro-organism ultimately isolated from the infected prosthesis (Surin, et al. 1983). These results have been confirmed by other studies (Pulido, et al. 2008, Wilson, et al. 1990). Bengston et al highlighted the significance of skin infections in haematogenous seeding of the prosthesis. One third of patients with haematogenous seeding in this cohort had concurrent or preceding skin infections that were identified as the probable primary focus for the bacteraemia(Bengtson & Knutson 1991).

2.3 Microbiology

Staphylococcus species account for approximately half of all prosthetic joint infections; this includes *Staphylococcus aureus* and coagulase negative Staphylococcus species, both methicillin sensitive and resistant. Gram-negative bacilli infections and polymicrobial infections are the two next most common groups of pathogens described. Other gram-positive bacteria such as Streptococcus and Enterococcus species occur less commonly (Bengtson & Knutson 1991, Berbari, et al. 1998, Fitzgerald, et al. 1977, Moran, et al. 2007, Pandey, et al. 2000, Pulido, et al. 2008, Steckelberg & Osmon 2000). Importantly, in all series, a small number of cases meet the definition for prosthetic joint infection, and yet remain culture negative on standard microbiologic techniques.

Reference	1	2	3	4	5	6	7	8	9	
Total number of isolates	*112*	*248*	*81*	*578*	*63*	*462*	*357*	*42*	*112*	
Coagulase negative Staphylococcus	13	31	48	30	21	19	17	24	33	**27.3**
Staphylococcus aureus	23	21	14	23	38	22	42	19	17	**23.8**
Streptococcus spp	5	7	10	9	13	9	6	12	10.7	**9.4**
Enterococcus spp	3	6	7	3	0	1	3	10	6.3	**4.6**
Diptheroids	2	4	4	0.5	2	0.6	1	0	5.4	**2.6**
Gram-negative bacilli	6	28	0	6	11	8	5	29	16.1	**12.7**
Propionibacterium	0	0.4	3	1.5	0	0	0.3	2	0.9	**0.9**
Polymicrobial	33	0	12	12	6	19	15	0	0	**9.7**
Anaerobes	3	2	0	2	0	6	2	2	6.3	**3.0**
Other	1	4	0	2	0	3	0.3	19	2.7	**3.5**
Culture negative	5	0	0	11	10	12	8	2	1.8	**5.2**

1. (Moran, et al. 2007), 2. (Sharma, et al. 2008), 3. (Pandey, et al. 2000), 4. (Steckelberg & Osmon 2000), 5. (Pulido, et al. 2008), 6. (Berbari, et al. 1998), 7. (Bengtson & Knutson 1991), 8. (Fitzgerald, et al. 1977), 9. (McDonald, et al. 1989)

Table 1. Microbiological isolates in reported literature (percent)

3. Pathogenesis

3.1 Acquisition of infection

Acquisition of prosthetic joint infection occurs by two mechanisms: direct inoculation and haematogenous seeding. Direct inoculation of the prosthesis may occur at the time of implantation or with manipulation of the arthroplasty and is thought to be the predominant mechanism of infection. In a study by Southwood et al the 50% infective dose (ID_{50}) of *Staphylococcus aureus* required to induce infection with direct inoculation of the prosthesis was just 50 organisms. This compared to an intravenous inoculum dose of 100 000 organisms at the time of operation for bacteraemic seeding and infection of the prosthesis to occur. Southwood also demonstrated that three weeks after implantation of the prosthesis, the likelihood of bacteraemic seeding of the prosthesis was significantly reduced. In fact, in the rabbit model, the inoculum of intravenous bacteria required was near to the lethal dose(Southwood, et al. 1985). Nevertheless, haematogenous seeding remains an important cause of arthroplasty infections and it has been reported that up to 34% of patients with prosthetic joints in-situ developed deep infection of that prosthesis following an intercurrent episode of *Staphylococcus aureus* bacteraemia (Murdoch, et al. 2001).

Whilst theoretically distinct, clinically there is significant overlap between both mechanisms of infection. The simplified view is that infection resulting from inoculation occurs within the first year of implantation whilst haematogenous infections occur later. However the clinical presentation of prosthetic joint infections acquired during the original operation may be much more delayed, particularly with low virulence organisms such as coagulase negative staphylococcus species (Steckelberg & Osmon 2000). Furthermore, up to 50% of suspected prosthetic joint infections of haematogenous origin present within the first two years (Deacon, et al. 1996). However it is important to note that distinguishing between whether an episode of bacteraemia led to haematogenous seeding of a prosthetic joint or whether the primary source of the bacteraemia was a subclinical prosthetic joint infection can be problematic.

3.2 The role of biofilms

The pathogenesis of prosthetic joint infections is intimately connected to the property of biofilm formation by microorganisms. The presence of this biofilm can have a critical effect on the likely success of treatment for a number of reasons. Bacteria can exist in two unique forms; the free living or planktonic forms characterised by rapid cellular division, and the stationary or sessile forms characterised by slower cellular division (Costerton 1999, Costerton, et al. 1995).

The sessile bacteria secrete an extracellular matrix or slime. Together the microorganisms and this matrix comprise what is known as 'the biofilm'. The abiotic matrix performs a number of functions including provision of anchorage onto structures to support the sessile colonies(Donlan & Costerton 2002). It also facilitates communication between bacteria within the biofilm. This communication termed 'quorum sensing', is analogous to the paracrine signalling in multicellular organisms and enables the bacteria to regulate their gene synthesis(Gristina & Costerton 2009). Importantly, the matrix can provide bacteria with protection from antimicrobial chemicals and from host defense mechanisms. This impairment of host defense mechanisms has been demonstrated in a number of in vitro models. For example, the extracellular slime produced by *Staphylococcus epidermidis* can inhibit the phagocytic activity of neutrophils(Shiau & Wu 1998).

The concentration of antibiotic required to inhibit the growth of bacteria in biofilms is higher than that required to kill free-living bacteria. The mean inhibitory concentration (MIC) of many antibiotics is higher with the sessile forms than corresponding planktonic forms. Studies have demonstrated up to a 1000 fold increase in the MIC to particular antibiotics for bacteria moving from the planktonic to the sessile phenotype (Amorena, et al. 1999, Jones, et al. 2001, Rose & Poppens 2009, Schwank, et al. 1998, Souli & Giamarellou 1998, Stewart & Costerton 2001). This poses a major challenge for clinicians interpreting the reported antibiotic susceptibility results of bacteria, as our standard laboratory antibiotic susceptibility testing uses only the planktonic forms of bacteria. Newer technologies including the Calgary Biofilm Device can enable antibiotic susceptibility testing of the sessile phenotype of bacteria, but at present these are limited to a research setting and are not widely available(Ceri, et al. 1999).

There are a number of postulated mechanisms for the apparent resistance of biofilm residing bacteria to the effects of antibiotics. Firstly, the antibiotic may be deactivated at the surface of the biofilm. Secondly, the altered nutritional and biochemical environment within the biofilm may alter the activity of the antibiotics. Thirdly, antibiotics, particular cell wall active antibiotics such as betalactam antibiotics, rely on rapid growth and reproduction of the microorganism for their effect. These antibiotics are effective against the planktonic phenotype but have limited efficacy against the sessile phenotype as cellular turnover is greatly reduced. Finally the sessile forms act as 'spore-like' structures, which may act as a nidus for later relapse of infection (Costerton 1999, Stewart & Costerton 2001, Trampuz, et al. 2003, Zimmerli 2006).

The properties of the biofilm alter with time; with age many biofilms become increasingly resistant to antibiotics. Monzon et al demonstrated the efficacy of vancomycin against *Staphylococcus epidermidis* decreased as a biofilm aged. This phenomenon was not consistent with all antibiotics; the activity of rifampicin and tetracyclines was not altered (Monzon, et al. 2002). Using Ribosomal RNA Fluorescence In Situ Hybridization studies, Poulson et al assessed the growth rate of biofilms and demonstrated that the cellular turnover was significantly higher in younger biofilms compared to established biofilms (Poulsen, et al. 1993). This finding could account for the difference to antimicrobial susceptibility observed. Implant factors are also recognised to play a role in the pathogenesis of infection. Biochemical properties of prosthetic material influences bacterial adhesion and may impair host immune responses. For example, methyl methacrylate cement has been shown to inhibit complement and lymphocyte activity (Panush & Petty 1978, Petty 1978).

4. Diagnosis

4.1 Clinical features

The clinical diagnosis of prosthetic joints is challenging. Many typical symptoms of infection are often absent. Pain is the predominant symptom of prosthetic joint infections and is present in 90 to 100% of patients. The presence of fever is variable with 9 to 43% of patients in most case series having documented elevated temperatures (Canner, et al. 1984, Inman, et al. 1984, McDonald, et al. 1989, Miley, et al. 1982, Morrey, et al. 1989, Windsor, et al. 1990). In acute infections, erythema and swelling of the joint are often present, but are less common in more chronic infections (Del Pozo & Patel 2009, Miley, et al. 1982, Zimmerli, et al. 2004). A discharging sinus is associated with chronic, indolent presentations (Del Pozo & Patel 2009).

Zimmerli et al classifies arthroplasty infections as: Early (developing in the first three months after surgery), Delayed (occurring three to 24 months after surgery) and Late (greater than 24 months). This classification roughly correlates to important observed differences in the causative pathogens; with virulent organisms such as *Staphylococcus aureus* characteristically presenting earlier and more indolent pathogens such as coagulase negative Staphylococcus usually presenting later (Zimmerli, et al. 2004).

4.2 Laboratory studies

Peripheral blood leucocytosis is a poor predictor of infected arthroplasty; less than 10% of patients with an infected prosthesis have an elevated white cell count in most series (Canner, et al. 1984, Inman, et al. 1984, Zimmerli, et al. 2004). Other biochemical tests, such as the erythrocyte sedimentation rate (ESR) and C-reactive protein (CRP) are more useful diagnostic tests for these infections. For patients with proven infection of knee or hip arthroplasty, the ESR had a sensitivity of 81-92% and a specificity of 90-96%, while the CRP had a sensitivity of 84-89% and a specificity of 83-96% (Bottner, et al. 2007, Spangehl, et al. 1999). There are however, limitations to the diagnostic utility of the ESR and CRP. These markers are normally elevated after primary uncomplicated arthroplasty; the ESR peaks in the first week and may remain elevated for up to a year, while the CRP peaks at day 2 and may remain elevated for 3 weeks (Aalto, et al. 1984, Larsson, et al. 1992, Shih, et al. 1987).

The search for other biochemical markers of infection has included interleukin 6 (Il-6), tumour necrosis factor α (TNF-α) and procalcitonin C. Il-6 and TNF-α are cytokines released by monocytes and macrophages in the setting of infection (Bottner, et al. 2007). Procalcitonin is a precursor of calcitonin, and has been shown to be a specific marker of bacterial sepsis (Fernandez Lopez, et al. 2003). In a review by Bottner et al of 78 patients undergoing revision arthroplasties Il-6, TNF-α and procalcitonin were all significantly elevated in patients with confirmed septic loosening. The sensitivity and specificity respectively of Il-6 was 95% and 87%, TNF-α 43% and 94% and procalcitonin 33% and 98%. (Bottner, et al. 2007). Il-6 is elevated in the post-operative period for primary arthroplasty however, in a study by Shah et al, Il-6 was shown to return to normal levels within 2 days of the operation. Therefore there is potential diagnostic utility of Il-6 over CRP and ESR in the early post-operative period if infection is suspected, particularly in the first 21 days (Shah, et al. 2009).

Synovial fluid characteristics can be used to assist in diagnosis of prosthetic joint infections. In a study by Trampuz and colleagues, the leucocyte count was significantly higher in patients with prosthetic joint infection with a median of $18.9 \times 10^3/\mu L$ (range, 0.3 to 178 x $10^3/\mu L$) compared to a median leucocyte count of $0.3 \times 10^3/\mu L$ (range, 0.1 to 16 x $10^3/\mu L$) in patients with aseptic loosening. Using receiver operating characteristic (ROC) curves the authors found a synovial total white cell count $1.7 \times 10^3/\mu L$ and a leucocyte differential of greater than 65% neutrophils had a sensitivity and specificity of 94%, 88% and 97%, 98% respectively (Trampuz, et al. 2004).

4.3 Radiological studies

Plain radiographs lack sensitivity and specificity in diagnosing septic arthroplasty. Findings such as lucency around the prosthesis can be noted in both septic and aseptic loosening situations (Figure 1 A-D). In early infection plain radiographs are frequently normal (Miller 2005).

Technetium-Methylene Diphosphonate (MDP) bone scintigraphy is a sensitive test for prosthetic joint infection (Figure 1 E-G), but lacks specificity, as it does not differentiate between aseptic and septic loosening(Ghanem, et al. 2009). The bone scan can also remain positive for a year following primary arthroplasty. Bone scan does have a high negative predictive value therefore bone scans potentially can be used to exclude infection in the setting of a painful prosthetic joint (Smith, et al. 2001). Similar findings have been documented with newer modalities such as ^{18}F-Fluoro-deoxyglucose positron emission tomography (FDG-PET) (Delank, et al. 2006, Zoccali, et al. 2009). A recent meta-analysis of FDG-PET reported a sensitivity of 82.1% and specificity of 86.6% for the presence of prosthetic joint infection, and hence this may be a useful test if available(Kwee, et al. 2008).

Computer tomography (CT) and magnetic resonance imaging are not considered useful imaging modalities due to artefact from the metal prosthesis interfering with interpretation of imaging findings. However newer CT scanners can minimise this effect and may be useful in detecting abnormalities of the soft tissues in periprosthetic infections (Figure 2 A-E) but do not diagnose periprosthetic bone abnormalities well (Cyteval, et al. 2002)

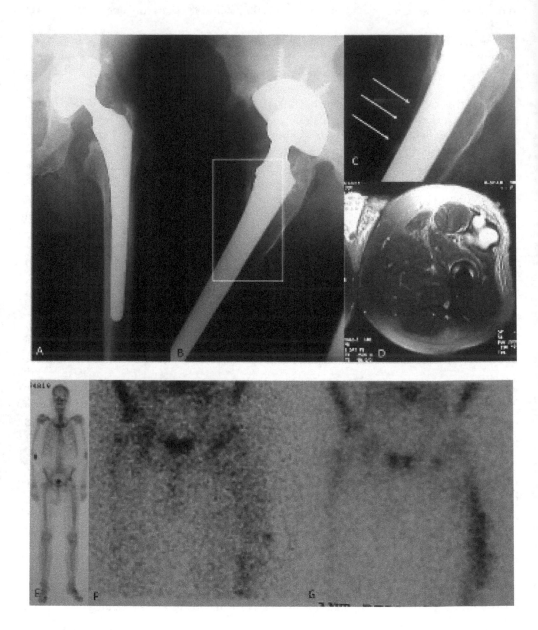

Fig. 1. (A) Painful (left) cementless hip prosthesis in situ. (B) Note extrinsic scalloping of anterior cortex of femoral diaphysis (box). (C) Magnified image of anterior femoral cortex with extrinsic scalloping (arrows) caused by soft tissue abscess (D). (E) Nuclear bone scan (TcMDP) demonstrating mild uptake over left proximal femur. Indium white cell scan at (F) 4 hours and (G) showing marked retention of nuclear tracer at 20 hours.

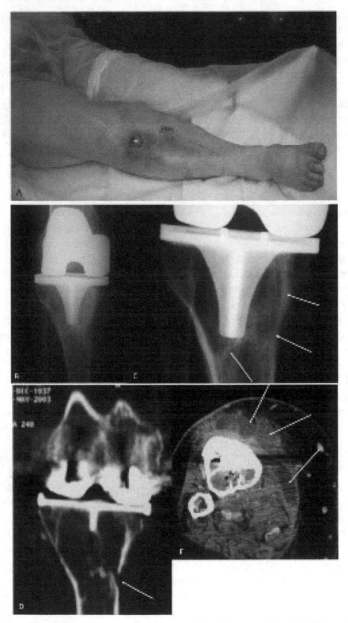

Fig. 2. (A) Localised infective sinus at the centre of incision used for total knee joint replacement. (B) plain radiograph showing periprosthetic sclerosis and lysis under the tibial component. (C) Magnified image showing obvious periprosthetic lysis (arrows). (D) Computer tomogram showing lysis under tibial component extending through medial cortex as cloaca (arrow). (E) Computer tomogram demonstrating soft tissue abscess formation (arrows) in continuity with intramedullary suppuration.

4.4 Histopathology diagnosis

Intraoperative frozen section histopathologic studies of periprosthetic tissue can be used as an adjunctive test for the diagnosis of prosthetic joint infections. An early paper showed a correlation between the polymorphonuclear leucocyte (PMN) count in tissue on histopathologic examination and the diagnosis of infection (Mirra, et al. 1976). Subsequent studies using frozen section histopathology for revision arthroplasty (using a PMN count of five to ten cells per high power field to diagnose infection) had a sensitivity of 50-93% and sensitivity of 77-100% (Bori, et al. 2006, Frances Borrego, et al. 2007, Ko, et al. 2005, Nunez, et al. 2007). It should be noted that inflammatory conditions such as rheumatoid arthritis may also cause a high PMN count, hence lowering specificity (Mirra, et al. 1976).

4.5 Microbiology diagnosis

The identification of the causative pathogen in a prosthetic device infection is of paramount importance. It allows for the institution of appropriate management strategies for infection including selection of the most appropriate antibiotic to target the pathogen, while minimising unnecessary antibiotic overuse, thus decreasing the incidence of drug toxicity and generally permitting simpler drug regimens to improve patient adherence.

It has earlier been noted that culture negative prosthetic joint infections continue to occur. Recent studies have focused on methods to increase the sensitivity of microbiological diagnostic techniques to address this problem. In a prospective study, which aimed to establish microbiological criteria for the diagnosis of prosthetic joint infection in revision arthroplasty, Atkins et al found that the isolation of indistinguishable microorganisms from three or more periprosthetic tissue samples has a sensitivity of 65% and a specificity of 99.6% for prosthetic joint infection. Utilising mathematical modelling the authors recommended that five to six intraoperative specimens of periprosthetic tissue be obtained to optimise the likelihood of a microbiologic diagnosis in prosthetic joint infection. They also noted that routine gram staining of periprosthetic tissue at revision arthroplasty had a very low sensitivity (12%) and the authors recommended that gram stain should be abandoned in revision arthroplasty cases, instead relying on culture (Atkins, et al. 1998).

Prolonged cultures may also help to improve the diagnostic yield. An increase in positive culture results of 24.6% when culture incubation of periprosthetic tissue samples was increased from 3 to fourteen days has been reported and in particular the isolation of fastidious organisms, such as Propionibacterium species was increased (Schafer, et al. 2008).

A number of techniques have been developed in an attempt to disrupt the biofilm and increase the yield of microbiological cultures. One such technique is ultrasonification whereby the explanted prosthesis is placed in a sterile polyethylene bag then in a sterile anaerobic jar, Ringer's solution is added and sonication is performed. The sonicate fluid is cultured aerobically and anaerobically. One study comparing sonication to standard tissue culture involving 331 patients of whom 79 had prosthetic joint infections; sonication yielded an additional 14 microbiological diagnosis with a reported sensitivity of 78.5% and specificity of 98.8%. The authors noted that sonication was particularly useful in cases where patients had received antibiotics perioperatively (Trampuz, et al. 2007).

4.6 Molecular techniques

Newer molecular techniques have been applied to prosthetic joint infections to increase the diagnostic yield including polymerase chain reaction (PCR), fluorescent in situ hybridization (FISH) and immunofluorescent microscopy (IFM). Both PCR and FISH target specific regions of bacterial genetic material, commonly bacterial ribosomal RNA (rRNA). The advantage of using rRNA is that it is highly conserved in bacterial species compared to most protein encoding genes. Both methods can use broad range oligonucleotide primers or more targeted primers including genus and species specific primers (Amann & Fuchs 2008).

A number of studies investigating the role of bacterial 16s rRNA PCR have been performed. Sensitivities of this technique ranged from 63-100% in detecting bacteria involved in prosthetic joint infection (De Man, et al. 2009, Hoeffel, et al. 1999, Mariani, et al. 1996, Moojen, et al. 2007). In a study by Mariani et al 50 patients with symptoms following total knee arthroplasty underwent synovial fluid and intraoperative tissue sampling for culture and PCR; cultures were positive in fifteen specimens compared to 32 specimens when PCR was applied (Mariani, et al. 1996). Likewise Tunney et al used PCR in a study of 120 patients undergoing prosthetic hip joint revision. The explanted prosthesis underwent ultrasonification and this fluid was cultured and underwent 16s DNA PCR. Standard microbiologic cultures were positive in 22% of patients, compared to 72% of patients with positive results from PCR (Tunney, et al. 1999). The limitation of these studies was a paucity of correlation with clinical or histological features of infection. In a review of 34 patients with confirmed prosthetic joint infection Vandercam et al found that PCR was positive in 31 of 34 patients (91.2%), compared to positive microbiological culture in 22 of 34 patients (64.7%). Of import, eight of the nine patients with positive PCR but negative culture results had received antibiotic therapy in the prior ten days (Vandercam, et al. 2008). Despite these promising results, the weakness of 16s ribosomal RNA PCR techniques is the low specificity and high false positive rate. In a study by Clarke et al 29% of the patients without septic arthritis (on the basis of clinical, radiological, biochemical, intraoperative findings, culture and histology) had positive PCR results, this was particularly pronounced in the cohort undergoing revision arthroplasty for aseptic loosening where 46% of patients had positive PCR (Clarke, et al. 2004). The high false positive rate may be due to a number of factors including contamination of specimen or the reagents and detection of necrotic bacterial DNA (Bauer, et al. 2006). Importantly though, many patients labelled as having aseptic loosening may in fact have had low grade chronic infection contributing to prosthesis loosening. Given that there is no gold standard to define prosthetic joint infection, the specificity of PCR remains difficult to judge.

FISH is a technique that uses labelled oligonucleotide probes that hybridise to specific genetic regions on bacteria and are subsequently visualised using fluorescent microscopy or flow cytometry (Amann & Fuchs 2008, Moter & Gobel 2000). Probes to detect bacterial rRNA or other genetic targets are available and these include species specific probes, therefore allowing identification and simultaneous observation of the different bacteria. FISH also allows an appreciation of the architectural arrangement of the organisms within the biofilm which can assist in differentiating true infections from contamination (McDowell & Patrick 2005, Moter & Gobel 2000). In orthopaedic infections it has been demonstrated that *Staphylococcus aureus* and *Staphylococcus epidermidis* could be visualised and differentiated in an experimental biofilm. Additionally, in a clinical case of septic loosening of a hip prosthesis, *Staphylococcus epidermidis* was visualised using FISH techniques in periprosthetic tissue samples(Krimmer, et al. 1999). FISH has otherwise not yet been widely applied to prosthetic joint infections in a clinical setting.

Immunofluorescence microscopy (IFM) is another novel nonculture technique for diagnosing prosthetic joint infections. In immunofluorescence microscopy, samples are mixed with monoclonal antibodies (MAb) to specific antigens on bacterial cell walls. Samples are then incubated with a second antibody conjugated with a fluorescent dye. The bacteria are then visualised using fluorescence microscopy(Tunney, et al. 1999). As with FISH, IFM can be used to assess the biofilm structure and can detect multiple pathogens (McDowell & Patrick 2005, Tunney, et al. 1999). In the study by Tunney et al IFM was performed on the sonicate fluid from explanted prostheses using Mab for both Propionibacterium and Staphylococcus species. (Tunney, et al. 1999).

5. Treatment

5.1 Treatment goal

Optimal treatment of prosthetic joint infections involves the eradication of infection whilst maintaining function of the joint and patient quality of life (Zimmerli, et al. 2004). However there are no large, multi-centred, randomised prospective studies of treatment strategies to guide recommendations. The successful treatment of prosthetic joints is contingent on the elimination of the biofilm dwelling microorganism. The two mainstay methods of achieving this are through either surgical removal of the prosthesis or through use of biofilm active antibiotics in conjunction with surgical debridement and retention of the prosthesis.

The surgical strategies used to treat arthroplasty infections include: resection arthroplasty, one-stage or two-stage exchange procedures, amputation and debridement and retention. Resection arthroplasty entails the removal of all foreign material including cement, resection of devitalised tissue and bone and may or may not involve arthrodesis. Exchange procedures involve resection arthroplasty with reimplantation of a new joint prosthesis performed at the time of removal of the infected prosthesis (one-stage exchange); or delayed by a variable period of time while antibiotic therapy is administered (two-stage exchange). Debridement and retention of the prosthesis usually involves open arthrotomy, removal of all infected and necrotic bone, exchange of liners and lavage of the joint (Giulieri, et al. 2004, Matthews, et al. 2009, Rand, et al. 1986, Steckelberg & Osmon 2000, Trampuz & Zimmerli 2008, Zimmerli, et al. 2004).

A number of factors influence the surgical approach selected for an individual patient, these include a patient's general health and fitness for anaesthesia, condition of the prosthesis and bone stock, the causative agent, the timing of the infection relative to the prosthesis insertion, the availability of effective antibiotics and clinicians' and patient preference.

5.2 Systemic antibiotic therapy without surgical debridement

Administration of antibiotic therapy without surgical management is not routinely recommended, as it is rarely associated with successful cure. Early studies of antibiotic therapy alone for prosthetic joint infections had disappointing results with successful outcomes in as little as 8-15% of patients (Bengtson, et al. 1989, Canner, et al. 1984). The confounding factor when analysing these poor results is that biofilm active antibiotics, were not used. Treatment with biofilm active antibiotics alone including rifampicin and ciprofloxacin for three to six months has yielded successful outcomes in highly selected patients; those presenting with early infections (less than one year following implant), infection due to *Staphylococcus aureus*, absence of implant loosening and strict adherence to treatment (Trebse, et al. 2005). However, antibiotic suppression alone is generally reserved for patients with significant comorbidities in whom surgery is contraindicated, who are without evidence of systemic infection and where tolerable oral antibiotics are available. Given the low likelihood of cure, many clinicians view this as long term, often lifelong suppressive therapy, embarked upon without curative intent (Steckelberg & Osmon 2000, Zimmerli, et al. 2004).

5.3 Exchange arthroplasty

Interpretation of the current literature describing the outcomes of patients having one- and two-stage exchange procedures is challenging owing to the heterogeneity of the patient populations, the causative organisms and the surgical techniques (including use of antibiotic impregnated cement), the differences in the duration of patient follow up and probable publication bias. The greatest concern with one-stage exchange procedures is the implantation of the prosthesis into an infected field with subsequent reinfection of the revised arthroplasty. In one-stage exchange, reported success rates range from 38-100%; but there is significant variability in the definition of success which includes freedom from infection, freedom from pain or simply the presence of a functional joint (Callaghan, et al. 1999, Jamsen, et al. 2009, Steckelberg & Osman 2000). In examination of the outcomes of one-stage exchange revision hip arthroplasty, 80% (range 57-92%) of patients have been reported to remain infection free after one-stage exchange without the use of antibiotic cement (Steckelberg & Osman 2000). When antibiotic impregnated cement was used, 88% (range 76-100%) of patients have been reported to remain infection free at follow up (Callaghan, et al. 1999, Jackson & Schmalzried 2000, Langlais 2003, Steckelberg & Osman 2000). Results for one-stage exchange in knee arthroplasty revision are in general worse than for hips, with only 65% (range 57-100%) of patients remaining free of recurrence of infection at follow up (Steckelberg & Osmon 2000). On the basis of these results, one-stage exchange of an infected prosthesis is rarely advised for prosthetic knee infections(Trampuz & Zimmerli 2008, Zimmerli, et al. 2004). There are, however some advantages with one-stage exchange; patients undergo a single operation and generally require a shorter period of hospitalisation in total.

Consensus recommendations for one-stage exchange suggest that it should only be considered where there is minimal soft tissue damage and where less virulent organisms are involved (Hirakawa, et al. 1998, Jackson & Schmalzried 2000, Miley, et al. 1982, Trampuz & Zimmerli 2008, Zimmerli, et al. 2004). The presence of sinus tract is considered a relative contraindication for one-stage exchange. Ideally the causative agent should be known prior to resection arthroplasty and treatment commenced preoperatively(Zimmerli, et al. 2004).

In two-stage exchange procedures, reimplantation is delayed for a variable length of time from 2 weeks to several months. Spacers impregnated with antibiotic are commonly inserted to maintain limb length and improve patient mobility during that interval (Leunig, et al. 1998). Antibiotics with activity against the isolated pathogen are administered for at least 6 weeks. Tissue samples are often routinely taken from the periprosthetic tissue at the time of reimplantation for microbiological culture to assess the efficacy of the interim treatment (Insall, et al. 1983, Wilson, et al. 1990, Windsor, et al. 1990). In infections with difficult-to-treat micro-organisms such as MRSA, resistant enterococci and fungi, current consensus guidelines recommends prolonged interval between removal and reimplantation without the use of a spacer (Trampuz & Zimmerli 2008, Zimmerli, et al. 2004)

Two-stage exchange, in general, has a higher success rate compared to one-stage with rates of 63-100% (Colyer & Capello 1994, Haleem, et al. 2004, Jamsen, et al. 2009, Woods, et al. 1983). In hip arthroplasty two-stage exchange without the use of antibiotic impregnated cement, 81% of patients (range 53-100%) remain free of recurrent infection increasing to 93% (73-100%) when antibiotic cement is used (Laffer, et al. 2006, Langlais, et al. 2006, Steckelberg & Osman 2000). In knee arthroplasty infections, 84% (38-100%) of patients in whom antibiotic cement is not used, and 88% (63-100%) of patients in whom antibiotic impregnated cement is used remain infection free following two stage exchange (Bengtson, et al. 1989, Grogan, et al. 1986, Hanssen, et al. 1994, Insall, et al. 1983, Morrey, et al. 1989, Rand, et al. 1986, Wang & Chen 1997, Wasielewski, et al. 1996, Wilson, et al. 1990, Windsor, et al. 1990, Woods, et al. 1983).

A number of factors potentially influence treatment outcomes in two-stage exchange procedures. Polymicrobial infection, infection with virulent organisms including *Staphylococcus aureus* and methicillin resistant coagulase negative Staphylococcus species, the presence of rheumatoid arthritis and a history of prior multiple revisions have all been shown to associated with lower rates of success in two-stage exchanges (Hirakawa, et al. 1998, Lim, et al. 2009, Mittal, et al. 2007). Current consensus guidelines recommend two-stage exchange in chronic infections with moderately or severely damaged tissue or if a sinus tract is present (Trampuz & Zimmerli 2008, Zimmerli, et al. 2004).

5.4 Resection arthroplasty

Resection arthroplasty and amputation are generally reserved for patients with refractory infections particularly where there is severe loss of bone stock or where functional improvement following revision is unlikely (Trampuz & Zimmerli 2008, Zimmerli, et al. 2004). Whilst rates of recurrence of infection are low, patients have worse functional outcomes and up to 80% of patients report residual pain following resection (Morrey, et al. 1989).

5.5 Debridement and retention of the prosthesis

Debridement and retention of the prosthesis is an attractive treatment option for many patients given that it is the least invasive, with a lower surgical morbidity, and is generally associated with good functional outcomes (Trampuz & Zimmerli 2008, Zimmerli, et al. 2004). Open arthrotomy and debridement is recommended when attempting retention of the prosthesis as poorer results are reported with arthroscopic 'washout' compared to open 'washout'(Laffer, et al. 2006). Following debridement, patients should receive biofilm active antibiotics generally for a longer duration than with surgical exchange or resection.

Early studies of debridement and prosthesis retention strategies to treat prosthetic joint infection were disappointing with recurrence of infection at 2 years reported in 69% of patients (Brandt, et al. 1997). Poor outcomes have been reported when symptoms are present greater than 8 days, when a sinus tract is present and with late chronic infections; In some instances all patients with late infection experienced treatment failure (Berbari, et al.

2006a, Crockarell, et al. 1998, Marculescu, et al. 2006b). High failure rates have also observed with specific organisms, only 12% of patients with *Staphylococcus aureus* infection experiencing successful treatment outcomes (Deirmengian, et al. 2003, Marculescu, et al. 2006a). Gram-negative infections, polymicrobial infections and culture negative prosthetic joint infections were also associated with higher rates of recurrence of infection following debridement and retention (Berbari, et al. 2007, Hsieh, et al. 2009a, Marculescu & Cantey 2008). However, successful outcomes have been reported in the setting of early or haematogenous infections (Morrey, et al. 1989, Wasielewski, et al. 1996). Tsuyakama et al reported a successful outcome in 71% of patients with early infections treated with debridement of the prosthetic joint followed by four weeks of parenteral antibiotics with an average follow up of 3.8 years (Tsukayama, et al. 1996).

Newer treatment strategies evolved as understanding of the role of biofilm in the pathogenesis of prosthetic joint infections increased. In vivo studies using guinea pig tissue-cage animal model by Widmer et al demonstrated the clinical utility of rifampicin in chronic biofilm infections (Widmer, et al. 1990). Further studies also identified that quinolones retained activity in the presence of biofilms (Schwank, et al. 1998, Widmer, et al. 1991).

The addition of rifampicin to antimicrobial regimens has led to a significant improvement in success rates reported in the treatment of gram-positive prosthetic joint infection; in many instances comparable to that reported for two-stage exchange. In our experience combination treatment including rifampicin has resulted in successful treatment in up to 90% of patients (Aboltins, et al. 2007); however successful outcomes are associated with several factors. Higher success rates are reported where the causative organism is a staphylococcus species and when antibiotic therapy is continued for a protracted period; 12 months or greater, (Choong, et al. 2007, Widmer, et al. 1992). In contrast the rate of success is significantly diminished when a fistula is present, particularly in knee arthroplasty where successful outcomes have been reported in only 45-69% of patients. (Drancourt, et al. 1993).

The only randomised double-blinded control trial examining the role of rifampicin in the treatment of prosthetic device staphylococcal infections was conducted from 1992 through 1997. The study involved 33 patients with orthopaedic device infections and duration of symptoms less than one year. Patients were randomised to receive rifampicin 450mg and ciprofloxacin 750mg (twice daily) or ciprofloxacin and placebo. Rifampicin/ciprofloxacin combination was successful in all patients compared to 58% of patients who received ciprofloxacin alone (Zimmerli, et al. 1998). Subsequent studies corroborated these results with success rates of greater than 85% of patients treated with debridement and retention and rifampicin containing antibiotic treatment (Berdal, et al. 2005, Byren, et al. 2009, Rao, et al. 2003). The main limitations with the use of rifampicin are the high likelihood of generation of resistance when used without a second antibiotic and the hepatic and gastrointestinal toxicities (John, et al. 2009, Widmer, et al. 1990). Therefore careful, regular follow up of patients is necessary and the management these antibiotics should involve collaboration between Infectious Diseases Physicians and Orthopaedic Surgeons.

The investigation of newer agents for the treatment of prosthetic joint infection is ongoing. In guinea pig foreign-body infection model, John et al assessed the activity of newer agents including linezolid and daptomycin, alone and in combination with rifampicin. In this study neither daptomycin nor linezolid had activity against adherent MRSA when used as monotherapy. When used in combination with rifampicin, daptomycin at a dose of 30mg/kg (corresponding to a dose of 6mg/kg in humans) cured 67% of cage infections. At this dose, no cases of rifampicin resistance emerged. Results were less encouraging for linezolid; even in combination with rifampicin, linezolid failed to cure any cage infection. Resistance to rifampicin emerged in 8% of cage infections treated with rifampicin-linezolid combinations (John, et al. 2009).

For gram-negative infections, ciprofloxacin has been shown to be effective in guinea pig tissue cage models(Widmer, et al. 1991). In a study of 28 patients with bone and joint infections secondary to gram-negative bacilli combination therapy with cefepime and fluoroquinolone obtained a cure in 79% of patients. However only 5 patients in this cohort had a prosthetic joint infection, two were treated with debridement and retention and only one of which was cured (the second patient died from a cause unrelated to the infection)(Legout, et al. 2006). In prosthetic joint infection secondary to gram negative bacilli, debridement and retention has yielded a success rate as low as 27% (Hsieh, et al. 2009b). This contrasts with our results where by infection free survival at 2 years was 94% in gram-negative infections when fluoroquinolone was used in conjunction with debridement and retention (Aboltins, et al. 2011). Again this is in the setting of short duration of symptoms (median 7 days) and prolonged oral antibiotic treatment (median 12 months).

The duration of antibiotic after debridement and retention varies in reported clinical studies ranging from six months to greater than 4 years. In a study by Laffer et al there was no difference in outcome in patients receiving three to six months of antibiotics compared with greater than six months (91% v 87% success). In this study patients were followed up for a median duration of 28 (range, 2–193) months and 55% of infections were caused by Staphylococcus species(Laffer, et al. 2006). In accordance with consensus guidelines, debridement and retention of the prosthetic joint should be considered in patients with a short duration of symptoms in the absence of implant loosening and soft tissue damage where antibiotics with biofilm activity are available (Laffer, et al. 2006, Matthews, et al. 2009, Trampuz & Zimmerli 2008, Zimmerli, et al. 2004).

6. Conclusion

Prosthetic joint infections involve a complex interplay between the biofilm forming microorganisms, host responses and the implant. These infections are an uncommon but devastating complication of arthroplasty. However with given the ageing population the number of patients requiring arthroplasty is set to increase exponentially. Clinical investigation is imperative to increase understanding, improve diagnosis, optimise treatment and ultimately prevent prosthetic joint infections. While 2-stage exchanges remains the most reliable and consistent treatment option in terms of successful outcomes, the advent of more accurate diagnostic tools and combining the use of newer antibiotic agents with debridement and retention of the prosthetic joint should be considered a viable treatment option rather than an alternative. However this works best where a clear treatment protocol has been established, that targets patients at the earliest onset of symptoms, where debridement is aggressive and treatment involves is a combined approach between infectious Diseases Physicians and Orthopaedic Surgeons. Results at our institution attest to the success of such a protocol.

7. References

Aalto, K., Osterman, K., Peltola, H. & Rasanen, J. Change in Erythrocyte sedimentation rate and c-reactive protein after total hip arthorplasty. *Clinical Orthopaedics and Related Research* 184, 118-120 (1984).

Aboltins, C.A., Dowsey, M.M., Buising, K.L., Peel, T.N., Daffy, J.R., Choong, P.F. & Stanley, P.A. Gram-negative prosthetic joint infection treated with debridement, prosthesis retention and antibiotic regimens including a fluoroquinolone. *Clin Microbiol Infect* 17, 862-867 (2011).

Aboltins, C.A., Page, M.A., Buising, K.L., Jenney, A.W.J., Daffy, J.R. & Choong, P.F.M. Treatment of staphylococcal prosthetic joint infections with debridement , prosthesis retention and oral rifampicin and fusidic acid. *Clinical Microbiology and Infection* 13, 586-591 (2007).

Ahnfelt, L., Herberts, P., Malchau, H. & Andersson, G.B.J. Prognosis of total hip replacement. *Acta Orthopaedica Scandinavica* 61, 2-26 (1990).

Amann, R. & Fuchs, B.M. Single-cell identification in microbial communities by improved fluorescence in situ hybridization techniques. *Nature Reviews Microbiology* 6, 339-348 (2008).

Amorena, B., Gracia, E., Monzon, M., Leiva, J., Oteiza, C., Perez, M., Alabart, J.L. & Hernandez-Yago, J. Antibiotic susceptibility assay for Staphylococcus aureus in biofilms developed in vitro. *Journal of Antimicrobial Chemotherapy* 44, 43-55 (1999).

Atkins, B.L., Athanasou, N., Deeks, J.J., Crook, D.W.M., Simpson, H., Peto, T.E.A., Lardy-smith, P.M.C. & Berendt, A.R. Prospective Evaluation of Criteria for Microbiological Diagnosis of Prosthetic-Joint Infection at Revision Arthroplasty. *Journal of Clinical Microbiology* 36, 2932-2939 (1998).

Bauer, T.W., Parvizi, J., Kobayashi, N. & Krebs, V. Diagnosis of periprosthetic infection. *J Bone Joint Surg Am* 88-A, 869-882 (2006).

Bengtson, S. & Knutson, K. The infected knee arthroplasty. *Acta Orthopaedica Scandinavica* 62, 301-311 (1991).

Bengtson, S., Knutson, K. & Lidgren, L. Treatment of Infected Knee Arthroplasty. *Clinical Orthopaedics and Related Research* 245, 173-178 (1989).

Berbari, E.F., Hanssen, A.D., Duffy, M.C., Steckelberg, J.M., Ilstrup, D.M., Harmsen, W.S. & Osmon, D.R. Risk factors for prosthetic joint infection: case-control study. *Clin Infect Dis* 27, 1247-1254 (1998).

Berbari, E.F., Marculescu, C., Sia, I., Lahr, B.D., Hanssen, A.D., Steckelberg, J.M., Gullerud, R. & Osmon, D.R. Culture-negative prosthetic joint infection. *Clinical Infectious Diseases* 45, 1113-1119 (2007).

Berbari, E.F., Osmon, D.R., Duffy, M.C., Harmssen, R.N., Mandrekar, J.N., Hanssen, A.D. & Steckelberg, J.M. Outcome of prosthetic joint infection in patients with rheumatoid arthritis: the impact of medical and surgical therapy in 200 episodes. *Clinical Infectious Diseases* 42, 216-223 (2006a).

Berbari, E.F., Osmon, D.R., Duffy, M.C.T., Harmssen, R.N.W., Mandrekar, J.N., Hanssen, A.D. & Steckelberg, J.M. Outcome of prosthetic joint infection in patients with rheumatoid arthritis: the impact of medical and surgical therapy in 200 episodes. *Clinical Infectious Diseases* 42, 216-223 (2006b).

Berdal, J.E., Skramm, I., Mowinckel, P., Gulbrandsen, P. & Bjornholt, J.V. Use of rifampicin and ciprofloxacin combination therapy after surgical debridement in the treatment of early manifestation prosthetic joint infections. *Clinical Microbiology and Infection* 11, 843-845 (2005).

Bori, G., Soriano, A., GarcÃa, S.n., Gallart, X., Casanova, L., Mallofre, C., Almela, M., MartÃ-nez, J.a., Riba, J. & Mensa, J. Low sensitivity of histology to predict the presence of microorganisms in suspected aseptic loosening of a joint prosthesis. *Modern Pathology* 19, 874-877 (2006).

Bottner, F., Wegner, a., Winkelmann, W., Becker, K., Erren, M. & Gotze, C. Interleukin-6, procalcitonin and TNF-alpha: markers of peri-prosthetic infection following total joint replacement. *J Bone Joint Surg Am* 89-Br, 94-99 (2007).

Bozic, K.J. & Ries, M.D. The impact of infection after total hip arthroplasty on hospital and surgeon resource utilization. *J Bone Joint Surg Am* 87-A, 1746-1751 (2005).

Brandt, C.M., Sistrunk, W.W., Duffy, M.C., Hanssen, a.D., Steckelberg, J.M., Ilstrup, D.M. & Osmon, D.R. Staphylococcus aureus prosthetic joint infection treated with debridement and prosthesis retention. *Clinical Infectious Diseases* 24, 914-919 (1997).

Byren, I., Bejon, P., Atkins, B.L., Angus, B., Masters, S., McLardy-Smith, P., Gundle, R. & Berendt, a. One hundred and twelve infected arthroplasties treated with 'DAIR' (debridement, antibiotics and implant retention): antibiotic duration and outcome. *Journal of Antimicrobial Chemotherapy* 63, 1264-1271 (2009).

Callaghan, J.J., Katz, R.P. & Johnston, R.C. One-Stage Revision Surgery of the Infected Hip. *Clinical Orthopaedics and Related Research* 369, 139-143 (1999).

Canner, G.C., Steinberg, M.E., Heppenstall, R.B. & Balderston, R. The infected hip after total hip arthroplasty. *J Bone Joint Surg Am* 66-A, 1393-1399 (1984).

Ceri, H., Olson, M.E., Stremick, C., Read, R.R. & Morck, D. The Calgary Biofilm Device : New Technology for Rapid Determination of Antibiotic Susceptibilities of Bacterial Biofilms. *Journal of Clinical Microbiology* 37, 1771-1776 (1999).

Choong, P.F., Dowsey, M.M., Carr, D., Daffy, J. & Stanley, P. Risk factors associated with acute hip prosthetic joint infections and outcome of treatment with a rifampinbased regimen. *Acta Orthop* 78, 755-765 (2007).

Clarke, M.T., Roberts, C.P., Lee, P.T.H., Gray, J., Keene, G.S. & Rushton, N. Polymerase Chain Reaction Can Detect Bacterial DNA in Aseptically Loose Total Hip Arthroplasties. *Clinical Orthopaedics and Related Research* 427, 132-137 (2004).

Colyer, R.a. & Capello, W.N. Surgical Treatment of the Infected Hip Implant. *Clinical Orthopaedics and Related Research* 298, 75-79 (1994).

Costerton, J.W. Bacterial Biofilms: A Common Cause of Persistent Infections. *Science* 284, 1318-1322 (1999).

Costerton, J.W., Lewandowski, Z., Caldwell, D.E., Korber, D.R. & Lappin-scott, H.M. Microbial biofilms. *Annual Reviews of Microbiology* 49, 711-745 (1995).

Crockarell, J.R., Hanssen, A.D., Osmon, D.R. & Morrey, B.F. Treatment of Infection with Debridement and Retention of the Components following Hip Arthroplasty

Treatment of Infection with Debridement and Retention of the Components following Hip Arthroplasty. *J Bone Joint Surg Am* 80-A, 1306-1313 (1998).

Cyteval, C., Hamm, V., Sarrabere, M.P., Lopez, F.M., Maury, P. & Taourel, P. Painful infection at the site of hip prosthesis: CT imaging. *Radiology* 224, 477-483 (2002).

De Man, F.H.R., Graber, P., Luem, M., Zimmerli, W., Ochsner, P.E. & Sendi, P. Broad-range PCR in selected episodes of prosthetic joint infection. *Infection* 37, 292-294 (2009).

Deacon, J.M., Pagliaro, A.J., Zelicof, S.B. & Horowitz, H.W. Current concepts review. Prophylactic use of antibiotics for procedures after total joint replacement. *J Bone Joint Surg Am* 78-A, 1755-1770 (1996).

Deirmengian, C., Greenbaum, J., Lotke, P.A., Booth, R.E. & Lonner, J.H. Limited Success with Open Debridement and Retention of Components in the Treatment of Acute Staphylococcus Aureus Infections After Total Knee Arthroplasty. *Journal of Arthroplasty* 18, 22-26 (2003).

Del Pozo, J.L. & Patel, R. Infection Associated with Prosthetic Joints. *New England Journal of Medicine* 361, 787-794 (2009).

Delank, K.S., Schmidt, M., Michael, J.W.P., Dietlein, M., Schicha, H. & Eysel, P. The implications of 18F-FDG PET for the diagnosis of endoprosthetic loosening and infection in hip and knee arthroplasty: results from a prospective, blinded study. *BMC Musculoskeletal Disorders* 7, 20-20 (2006).

Donlan, R.M. & Costerton, J.W. Biofilms : Survival Mechanisms of Clinically Relevant Microorganisms. *Clinical Microbiology and Infection* 15, 167-193 (2002).

Dowsey, M.M. & Choong, P.F. Obesity is a major risk factor for prosthetic infection after primary hip arthroplasty. *Clin Orthop Relat Res* 466, 153-158 (2008).

Dowsey, M.M. & Choong, P.F. Obese diabetic patients are at substantial risk for deep infection after primary TKA. *Clin Orthop Relat Res* 467, 1577-1581 (2009).

Drancourt, M., Stein, A., Argenson, J.N., Zannier, A., Curvale, G. & Raoult, D. Oral rifampin plus ofloxacin for treatment of Staphylococcus-infected orthopedic implants. *Antimicrobial Agents and Chemotherapy* 37, 1214-1218 (1993).

Fernandez Lopez, A., Luaces Cubells, C., García Garcia, J.J. & Fernandez Pou, J. Procalcitonin in pediatric emergency departments for the early diagnosis of invasive bacterial infections in febrile infants: results of a multicenter study and utility of a rapid qualitative test for this marker. *The Pediatric Infectious Disease Journal* 22, 895-903 (2003).

Fitzgerald, R.H., Nolan, D.R., Ilstrup, D.M., E., R., Washington, J.A. & Coventry, M.B. Deep wound sepsis following total hip arthroplasty. *J Bone Joint Surg Am* 59-A, 847-847 (1977).

Frances Borrego, A., Martinez, F.M., Cebrian Parra, J.L., Graneda, D.S., Crespo, R.G. & Lopez-Duran Stern, L. Diagnosis of infection in hip and knee revision surgery: intraoperative frozen section analysis. *International Orthopaedics* 31, 33-37 (2007).

Ghanem, E., Antoci, V., Jr., Pulido, L., Joshi, A., Hozack, W. & Parvizi, J. The use of receiver operating characteristics analysis in determining erythrocyte sedimentation rate and C-reactive protein levels in diagnosing periprosthetic infection prior to revision total hip arthroplasty. *Int J Infect Dis* 13, e444-449 (2009).

Giulieri, S.G., Graber, P., Ochsner, P.E. & Zimmerli, W. Management of infection associated with total hip arthroplasty according to a treatment algorithm. *Infection* 32, 222-228 (2004).

Graves, S., Davidson D, de Steiger R & A., T. Australian Orthopaedic Association National Joint Replacement Registry. Annual Report 2009. Adelaide: Australian Orthopaedic Association. (Adelaide, 2010).

Gristina, A.G. & Costerton, J.W. Bacterial adherence to biomaterials and tissue . The significance of its role in clinical sepsis to Biomaterials. *J Bone Joint Surg Am* 67-A, 264-273 (2009).

Grogan, T.J., Dorey, F., Rollins, J. & Amstutz, H.C. Deep sepsis following total knee arthroplasty. Ten-year experience at the University of California at Los Angeles Medical Center. *J Bone Joint Surg Am* 68-A, 226-234 (1986).

Haleem, A.A., Berry, D.J. & Hanssen, A.D. Mid-Term to Long-Term Followup of Two-stage Reimplantation for Infected Total Knee Arthroplasty. *Clinical Orthopaedics and Related Research* 428, 35-39 (2004).

Hanssen, A.D., Rand, J.A. & Osmon, D.R. Treatment of the infected total knee arthroplasty with insertion of another prosthesis: the effect of antibiotic-impregnated bone cement. *Clinical Orthopaedics and Related Research*, 44-55 (1994).

Hirakawa, K., Stulberg, B.N., Wilde, A.H., Bauer, T.W. & Secic, M. Results of 2-stage reimplantation for infected total knee arthroplasty. *Journal of Arthoplasty* 13, 22-28 (1998).

Hoeffel, D.P., Hinrichs, S.H. & Garvin, K.L. Molecular diagnostics for the detection of musculoskeletal infection. *Clinical Orthopaedics and Related Research*, 37-46 (1999).

Horan, T.C., Gaynes, R.P., Martone, W.J., Jarvis, W.R. & Emori, G.T. CDC Definitions of Nosocomial Surgical Site Infections, 1992: A Modification of CDC Definitions of Surgical Wound Infections. *Infection Control and Hospital Epidemiology* 13, 606-608 (1992).

Hsieh, P.-H., Lee, M.S., Hsu, K.-Y., Chang, Y.-H., Shih, H.-N. & Ueng, S.W. Gram-negative prosthetic joint infections: risk factors and outcome of treatment. *Clinical Infectious Diseases* 49, 1036-1043 (2009a).

Hsieh, P.H., Lee, M.S., Hsu, K.Y., Chang, Y.H., Shih, H.N. & Ueng, S.W. Gram-negative prosthetic joint infections: risk factors and outcome of treatment. *Clin Infect Dis* 49, 1036-1043 (2009b).

Inman, R.D., Gallegos, K.V., Brause, B.D., Redecha, P.B. & Christian, C.L. Clinical and microbial features of prosthetic joint infection. *American Journal of Medicine* 77, 47-53 (1984).

Insall, J.N., Thompson, F.M. & Brause, B.D. Two-stage reimplantation for the salvage of infected total knee arthroplasty. *J Bone Joint Surg Am* 65-A, 1087-1087 (1983).

Jackson, W.O. & Schmalzried, T.P. Limited role of direct exchange arthroplasty in the treatment of infected total hip replacements. *Clinical Orthopaedics and Related Research* 381, 101-105 (2000).

Jamsen, E., Stogiannidis, I., Malmivaara, A., Pajamaki, J., Puolakka, T. & Konttinen, Y. Outcome of prosthesis exchange for infected knee arthroplasty: the effect of treatment approach. *Acta Orthopaedica* 80, 67-77 (2009).

John, A.-K., Baldoni, D., Haschke, M., Rentsch, K., Schaerli, P., Zimmerli, W. & Trampuz, A. Efficacy of daptomycin in implant-associated infection due to methicillin-resistant Staphylococcus aureus: importance of combination with rifampin. *Antimicrobial Agents and Chemotherapy* 53, 2719-2724 (2009).

Jones, S.M., Morgan, M., Humphrey, T.J. & Lappin-Scott, H. Effect of vancomycin and rifampicin on methicillin-resistant Staphylococcus aureus biofilms. *Lancet* 357, 40-41 (2001).

Ko, P., Ip, D., Chow, K., Cheung, F., Lee, O. & Lam, J. The Role of Intraoperative Frozen Section in Decision Making in Revision Hip and Knee Arthroplasties in a Local Community Hospital. *Journal of Arthoplasty* 20, 189-195 (2005).

Krimmer, V., Merkert, H., von Eiff, C., Frosch, M., Eulert, J., Lohr, J.F., Hacker, J. & Ziebuhr, W. Detection of Staphylococcus aureus and Staphylococcus epidermidis in clinical Samples by 16S rRNA-Directed In Site Hybridization. *Journal of Clinical Microbiology* 37, 2667-2673 (1999).

Kurtz, S., Ong, K., Lau, E., Mowat, F. & Halpern, M. Projections of primary and revision hip and knee arthroplasty in the United States from 2005 to 2030. *J Bone Joint Surg Am* 89-A, 780-785 (2007).

Kurtz, S.M., Lau, E., Schmier, J., Ong, K.L., Zhao, K. & Parvizi, J. Infection burden for hip and knee arthroplasty in the United States. *Journal of Arthoplasty* 23, 984-991 (2008).

Kurtz, S.M., Ong, K.L., Lau, E., Bozic, K.J., Berry, D. & Parvizi, J. Prosthetic joint infection risk after TKA in the Medicare population. *Clinical Orthopaedics and Related Research* 468, 52-56 (2010).

Kwee, T.C., Kwee, R.M. & Alavi, A. FDG-PET for diagnosing prosthetic joint infection: systematic review and metaanalysis. *European Journal of Nuclear Medicine and Molecular Imaging* 35, 2122-2132 (2008).

Laffer, R.R., Graber, P., Ochsner, P.E. & Zimmerli, W. Outcome of prosthetic knee-associated infection: evaluation of 40 consecutive episodes at a single centre. *Clin Microbiol Infect* 12, 433-439 (2006).

Langlais, F. Can we improve the results of revision arthroplasty for infected total hip replacement? *J Bone Joint Surg Am* 85-Br, 637-640 (2003).

Langlais, F., Belot, N., Ropars, M., Thomazeau, H., Lambotte, J.C. & Cathelineau, G. Antibiotic cements in articular prostheses: current orthopaedic concepts. *International Journal of Antimicrobial Agents* 28, 84-89 (2006).

Larsson, S., Thelander, U.L.F. & Friberg, S. C-reactive protein (CRP) levels after elective orthopedic surgery. *Clinical Orthopaedics and Related Research* 275, 237-242 (1992).

Legout, L., Senneville, E., Stern, R., Yazdanpanah, Y., Savage, C., Roussel-Delvalez, M., Rosele, B., Migaud, H. & Mouton, Y. Treatment of Bone and Joint Infections Caused by Gram-Nagative Bacilli with a Cefepime-Fluoroquinolone Combination. *Clinical Microbiology and Infection* 12, 1030-1033 (2006).

Leunig, M., Chosa, E., Speck, M. & Ganz, R. A cement spacer for two-stage revision of infected implants of the hip joint. *International Orthopaedics* 22, 209-214 (1998).

Lim, S.-j., Park, J.-c., Moon, Y.-w. & Park, Y.-s. Treatment of Periprosthetic Hip Infection Caused by Resistant Microorganisms Using 2-Stage Reimplantation Protocol. *Journal of Arthroplasty* 24, 1264-1269 (2009).

Marculescu, C.E., Berbari, E.F., Hanssen, A.D., Steckelberg, J.M., Harmsen, S.W., Mandrekar, J.N. & Osmon, D.R. Outcome of prosthetic joint infections treated with debridement and retention of components. *Clinical Infectious Diseases* 42, 471-478 (2006a).

Marculescu, C.E., Berbari, E.F., Hanssen, A.D., Steckelberg, J.M., Harmsen, S.W., Mandrekar, J.N. & Osmon, D.R. Outcome of prosthetic joint infections treated with debridement and retention of components. *Clinical Infectious Diseases* 42, 471-478 (2006b).

Marculescu, C.E. & Cantey, J.R. Polymicrobial Prosthetic Joint Infections. *Clinical Orthopaedics and Related Research* 466, 1397-1404 (2008).

Mariani, B.D., Martin, D.S., Levine, M.J., Booth, R.E. & Tuan, R.S. The Coventry Award. Polymerase chain reaction detection of bacterial infection in total knee arthroplasty. *Clinical Orthopaedics and Related Research*, 11-22 (1996).

Matthews, P.C., Berendt, a.R., McNally, M.a. & Byren, I. Diagnosis and management of prosthetic joint infection. *British Medical Journal* 338, b1773-b1773 (2009).

McDonald, D.J., Fitzgerald, R.H. & Ilstrup, D.M. Two-stage reconstruction of a total hip arthroplasty because of infection. *J Bone Joint Surg Am* 71-A, 828-834 (1989).

McDowell, A. & Patrick, S. Evaluation of Nonculture Methods for the Detection of Prosthetic Hip Biofilms. *Clinical Orthopaedics and Related Research* 437, 74-82 (2005).

Miley, G.B., Scheller, A.D. & Turner, R.H. Medical and surgical treatment of the septic hip with one-stage revision arthroplasty. *Clinical Orthopaedics and Related Research* 170, 76-76 (1982).

Miller, T.T. Imaging of knee arthroplasty. *European Journal of Radiology* 54, 164-177 (2005).

Mirra, J.M., Amstutz, H.C., Matos, M. & Gold, R. The pathology of the joint tissues and its clinical relevance in prosthesis failure. *Clinical Orthopaedics and Related Research* 117, 221-240 (1976).

Mittal, Y., Fehring, T.K., Hanssen, A., Marculescu, C., Odum, S.M. & Osmon, D. Two-stage reimplantation for periprosthetic knee infection involving resistant organisms. *J Bone Joint Surg Am* 89-A, 1227-1231 (2007).

Monzon, M., Oteiza, C., Leiva, J., Lamata, M. & Amorena, B. Biofilm testing of Staphylococcus epidermidis clinical isolates: low performance of vancomycin in relation to other antibiotics. *Diagnostic Microbiology and Infectious Disease* 44, 319-324 (2002).

Moojen, D.J.F., Spijkers, S.N.M., Schot, C.S., Nijhof, M.W., Vogely, H.C., Fleer, A., Verbout, A.J., Castelein, R.M., Dhert, W.J.a. & Schouls, L.M. Identification of orthopaedic infections using broad-range polymerase chain reaction and reverse line blot hybridization. *J Bone Joint Surg Am* 89-A, 1298-1305 (2007).

Moran, E., Masters, S., Berendt, A.R., McLardy-Smith, P., Byren, I. & Atkins, B.L. Guiding empirical antibiotic therapy in orthopaedics: The microbiology of prosthetic joint infection managed by debridement, irrigation and prosthesis retention. *Journal of Infection* 55, 1-7 (2007).

Morrey, B.F., Westholm, F., Schoifet, S., Rand, J.A. & Bryan, R.S. Long-Term Results of Various Treatment Options for Infected Total Knee Arthroplasty. *Clinical Orthopaedics and Related Research* 248 120-128 (1989).

Moter, A. & Gobel, U.B. Fluorescence in situ hybridization (FISH) for direct visualization of microorganisms. *Journal of Microbiological Methods* 41, 85-112 (2000).

Murdoch, D.R., Roberts, S.a., G., V., Shah, M.a., Taylor, S.L., Morris, a.J. & Corey, G.R. Infection of orthopedic prostheses after Staphylococcus aureus bacteremia. *Clinical Infectious Diseases* 32, 647-649 (2001).

Nunez, L.V., Buttaro, M.a., Morandi, A., Pusso, R. & Piccaluga, F. Frozen sections of samples taken intraoperatively for diagnosis of infection in revision hip surgery. *Acta Orthopaedica* 78, 226-230 (2007).

Ong, K.L., Kurtz, S.M., Lau, E., Bozic, K.J., Berry, D.J. & Parvizi, J. Prosthetic joint infection risk after total hip arthroplasty in the Medicare population. *Journal of Arthoplasty* 24, 105-109 (2009).

Pandey, R., Berendt, A.R. & Athanasou, N.A. Histological and microbiological findings in non-infected and infected revision arthroplasty tissues. *Archives of Orthopaedic and Trauma Surgery* 120, 570-574 (2000).

Panush, R.S. & Petty, R.W. Inhibition of human lymphocyte responses by methylmethacrylate. *Clinical Orthopaedics and Related Research* 134, 356-356 (1978).

Petty, W. The effect of methylmethacrylate on the bacterial inhibiting properties of normal human serum. *Clinical Orthopaedics and Related Research*, 266-278 (1978).

Poss, R., Thornhill, T.S., Ewald, F.C., Thomas, W.H., Batte, N.J. & Sledge, C.B. Factors influencing the incidence and outcome of infection following total joint arthroplasty. *Clinical Orthopaedics and Related Research* 182, 117-126 (1984).

Poulsen, L.K., Ballard, G. & Stahl, D.a. Use of rRNA fluorescence in situ hybridization for measuring the activity of single cells in young and established biofilms. *Applied and Environmental Microbiology* 59, 1354-1360 (1993).

Pulido, L., Ghanem, E., Joshi, A., Purtill, J.J. & Parvizi, J. Periprosthetic joint infection: the incidence, timing, and predisposing factors. *Clinical Orthopaedics and Related Research* 466, 1710-1715 (2008).

Rand, J.A., Bryan, R., Morrey, B. & Westholm, F. Management of Infected Total Knee Arthroplasty. *Clinical Orthopaedics and Related Research* 205, 75-85 (1986).

Rao, N., Crossett, L.S., Sinha, R.K. & L., J. Long-term suppression of infection in total joint arthroplasty. *Clinical Orthopaedics and Related Research* 414, 55-60 (2003).

Rose, W.E. & Poppens, P.T. Impact of biofilm on the in vitro activity of vancomycin alone and in combination with tigecycline and rifampicin against Staphylococcus aureus. *Journal of Antimicrobial Chemotherapy* 63, 485-488 (2009).

Schafer, P., Fink, B., Sandow, D., Margull, A., Berger, I. & Frommelt, L. Prolonged bacterial culture to identify late periprosthetic joint infection: a promising strategy. *Clinical Infectious Diseases* 47, 1403-1409 (2008).

Schwank, S., Rajacic, Z., Zimmerli, W. & Blaser, J. Impact of bacterial biofilm formation on in vitro and in vivo activities of antibiotics. *Antimicrobial Agents and Chemotherapyy* 42, 895-898 (1998).

Shah, K., Mohammed, A., Patil, S., McFadyen, A. & Meek, R.M.D. Circulating cytokines after hip and knee arthroplasty: a preliminary study. *Clinical Orthopaedics and Related Research* 467, 946-951 (2009).

Sharma, D., Douglas, J., Coulter, C., Weinrauch, P. & Crawford, R. Microbiology of infected arthroplasty: implications for empiric peri-operative antibiotics. *Journal of Orthopaedic Surgery (Hong Kong)* 16, 339-342 (2008).

Shiau, a.L. & Wu, C.L. The inhibitory effect of Staphylococcus epidermidis slime on the phagocytosis of murine peritoneal macrophages is interferon-independent. *Microbiology and Immunology* 42, 33-40 (1998).

Shih, L.-Y., Wu, J.-J. & Yanc, D.-J. Erythrocyte Sedimentation Rate and C-reactive Protein Values in Patients with Total Hip Arthroplasty. *Clinical Orthopaedics and Related Research* 225, 238-246 (1987).

Smith, S.L., Wastie, M.L. & Forster, I. Radionuclide bone scintigraphy in the detection of significant complications after total knee joint replacement. *Clinical radiology* 56, 221-224 (2001).

Souli, M. & Giamarellou, H. Effects of Slime Produced by Clinical Isolates of Coagulase-Negative Staphylococci on Activities of Various Antimicrobial Agents. *Antimicrobial Agents and Chemotherapy* 42, 939-941 (1998).

Southwood, R.T., Rice, J.L., McDonald, P.J., Hakendorf, P.H. & Rozenbilds, M.A. Infection in experimental hip arthroplasties. *J Bone Joint Surg Am* 67-Br, 229-231 (1985).

Spangehl, M.J., Masri, B.A., Connell, J.X.O. & Duncan, C.P. Prospective Analysis of Preoperative and Intraoperative Investigations for the Diagnosis of Infection at the Sites of Two Hundred and Two Revision Total Hip Arthroplasties. *J Bone Joint Surg Am* 81-A, 672-683 (1999).

Steckelberg, J.M. & Osman, D.R. Prosthetic Joint Infections. in *Infections Associated with Indwelling Medical Devices, 3rd ed.* (eds. Waldvogel, F.A. & Bisno, A.L.) 173-209 ASM Press, 1-55581-177-9, Washington D.C, 2000.

Steckelberg, J.M. & Osmon, D.R. Prosthetic Joint Infections. in *Infections Associated with Indwelling Medical Devices* (eds. Waldvogel, F.A. & Bisno, A.L.) 173-209 ASM Press, Washington DC, 2000.

Stewart, P.S. & Costerton, J.W. Antibiotic resistance of bacteria in biofilms. *Lancet* 358, 135-138 (2001).

Surin, V.V., Sundholm, K. & Backman, L. Infection After Total Hip Replacement. *Journal of Bone and Joint Surgery: British Volume* 65, 412-418 (1983).

Swan, J., Dowsey, M., Babazadeh, S., Mandaleson, A. & Choong, P.F. Significance of sentinel infective events in haematogenous prosthetic knee infections. *ANZ J Surg* 81, 40-45 (2011).

Trampuz, A., Hanssen, A.D., Osmon, D.R., Mandrekar, J., Steckelberg, J.M. & Patel, R. Synovial fluid leukocyte count and differential for the diagnosis of prosthetic knee infection. *American Journal of Medicine* 117, 556-562 (2004).

Trampuz, A., Osmon, D.R., Hanssen, A.D., Steckelberg, J.M. & Patel, R. Molecular and antibiofilm approaches to prosthetic joint infection. *Clinical Orthopaedics and Related Research*, 69-88 (2003).

Trampuz, A., Piper, K.E., Jacobson, M.J., Hanssen, A.D., Unni, K.K., Osmon, D.R., Mandrekar, J.N., Cockerill, F.R., Steckelberg, J.M., Greenleaf, J.F. & Patel, R. Sonication of removed hip and knee prostheses for diagnosis of infection. *New England Journal of Medicine* 357, 654-663 (2007).

Trampuz, A. & Zimmerli, W. Diagnosis and treatment of implant-associated septic arthritis and osteomyelitis. *Current Infectious Disease Reports* 10, 394-403 (2008).

Trebse, R., Pisot, V. & Trampuz, A. Treatment of infected retained implants. *J Bone Joint Surg Am* 87-Br, 249-256 (2005).

Tsukayama, D.T., Estrada, R. & Gustilo, R.B. Infection after total hip arthroplasty. A study of the treatment of one hundred and six infections. *J Bone Joint Surg Am* 78-A, 512-523 (1996).

Tunney, M.M., Patrick, S., Curran, M.D., Ramage, G., Hanna, D., Nixon, J.R., Gorman, S.P., Davis, R.I. & And, N. Detection of prosthetic hip infection at revision arthroplasty by immunofluorescence microscopy and PCR amplification of the bacterial 16S rRNA gene. *Journal of Clinical Microbiology* 37, 3281-3290 (1999).

Vandercam, B., Jeumont, S., Cornu, O., Yombi, J.-C., Lecouvet, F.d.r., LefÃ¨vre, P., Irenge, L.o.M. & Gala, J.-L. Amplification-based DNA analysis in the diagnosis of prosthetic joint infection. *Journal of Molecular Diagnostics* 10, 537-543 (2008).

Wang, J.W. & Chen, C.E. Reimplantation of infected hip arthroplasties using bone allografts. *Clinical Orthopaedics and Related Research* 335, 202-202 (1997).

Wasielewski, R.C., Barden, R.M. & Rosenberg, A.G. Results of different surgical procedures on total knee arthroplasty infections. *Journal of Arthoplasty* 11, 931-938 (1996).

Widmer, A.F., Frei, R., Rajacic, Z. & Zimmerli, W. Correlation between In Vivo and In Vitro Efficacy of Antimicrobial Agents against Foreign Body Infections. *Journal of Infectious Diseases* 162, 96-102 (1990).

Widmer, A.F., Gaechter, A., Ochsner, P.E. & Zimmerli, W. Antimicrobial treatment of orthopedic implant-related infections with rifampin combinations. *Clinical Infectious Diseases* 14, 1251-1253 (1992).

Widmer, A.F., Wiestner, A., Frei, R. & Zimmerli, W. Killing of Nongrowing and Adherent Escherichia coli Determines Drug Efficacy in Device-Related Infections. *Antimicrobial Agents and Chemotherapy* 35, 741-746 (1991).

Wilson, M.G., Kelley, K. & Thornhill, T.S. Infection as a complication of total knee-replacement arthroplasty. Risk factors and treatment in sixty-seven cases. *J Bone Joint Surg Am* 72-A, 878-883 (1990).

Windsor, R.E., Insall, J.N., Urs, W.K., Miller, D.V. & Brause, B.D. Two-stage reimplantation for the salvage of total knee arthroplasty complicated by infection. Further follow-up and refinement of indications. *J Bone Joint Surg Am* 72-A, 272-278 (1990).

Woods, G.W., Lionberger, D.R. & Tullos, H.S. Failed total knee arthroplasty: Revision and arthrodesis for infection and noninfectious complications. *Clinical Orthopaedics and Related Research* 173, 184-184 (1983).

Wymenga, A.B., van Horn, J.R., Theeuwes, A., Muytjens, H.L. & Slooff, T.J. Perioperative factors associated with septic arthritis after arthroplasty. Prospective multicenter study of 362 knee and 2,651 hip operations. *Acta Orthopaedica Scandinavica* 63, 665-671 (1992).

Yang, K., Yeo, S.J., Lee, B.P. & Lo, N.N. Total knee arthroplasty in diabetic patients: a study of 109 consecutive cases. *Journal of Arthoplasty* 16, 102-106 (2001).

Zimmerli, W. Prosthetic-joint-associated infections. *Best Practice and Research Clinical Rheumatology* 20, 1045-1063 (2006).

Zimmerli, W., Trampuz, A. & Ochsner, P.E. Prosthetic-joint infections. *New England Journal of Medicine* 351, 1645-1654 (2004).

Zimmerli, W., Widmer, A.F., Blatter, M., Frei, R. & Ochsner, P.E. Role of rifampin for treatment of orthopedic implant-related staphylococcal infections: a randomized controlled trial. *Journal of the American Medical Association* 279, 1537-1541 (1998).

Zoccali, C., Teori, G. & Salducca, N. The role of FDG-PET in distinguishing between septic and aseptic loosening in hip prosthesis: a review of literature. *International Orthopaedics* 33, 1-5 (2009).

3

Staphylococcus Infection Associated with Arthroplasty

Weisheng Ye, Wei Shang and Yaqiong Yang
Tianjin Orthopaedics Hospital
P. R. China

1. Introduction

Prosthetic joints improve the quality of life, but they may fail, necessitating revision or resection arthroplasty. The numbers of primary total hip and total knee arthroplasties have been increasing over the past decade, with nearly 800,000 such procedures performed in the United States in 2006 (Fig.1A)[1],with numbers projected to rise to 572,000 by 2030 and are expected to undergo a continuing rise, especially in light of an aging population[2]. Procedures to replace the shoulder, elbow, wrist, ankle, temporomandibular, metacarpophalangeal and interphalangeal joints are less commonly performed. The growth in the number of prosthetic joint replacement procedures provides new opportunities for infections to take hold.

The classification of the arthroplasty associated infection may distinguishes two major types—septic arthritis and osteomyelitis, which both involve the inflammatory destruction of joint and bone. The incidence of septic arthritis is between 2 and 10 in 100,000 in the general populace but may be as high as 30–70 per 100,000 in rheumatoid arthritis sufferers or recipients of prosthetic joints [3-5] and is more common in children than adults, and in males rather than females [6]. Haematogenous osteomyelitis most frequently effects children and the elderly [7]. In children, the incidence is typically between 1 in 5000 and 1 in 10,000 [8]. It has been argued that the incidence of haematogenous osteomyelitis is decreasing with an annual fall in childhood cases of 0.185 per 100,000 people recorded in Glasgow, Scotland between 1970 and 1997 [8-10]. Conversely, osteomyelitis resulting from direct infection is reportedly on the increase[10,11]. Local spread of infection from contiguous tissue to bone or direct infection can occur at any age, with foreign body implants a substantial risk factor [7].

Infection, although uncommon, is the most serious complication, occurring in 0.8 to 1.9% of knee arthroplasties[12-14] and 0.3 to 1.7% of hip arthroplasties[14-16]. The frequency of infection is increasing as the number of primary arthroplasties increases (Fig. 1B)[17]. These infections are increasingly difficult to treat with the rise in antibiotic-resistant forms.

2. Risk factors for infection

Patient-related risk factors for infection include previous revision arthroplasty or previous infection associated with a prosthetic joint at the same site, tobacco abuse, obesity, rheumatoid arthritis, a neoplasm, immunosuppression, and diabetes mellitus.

Surgical risk factors include simultaneous bilateral arthroplasty, a long operative time(>2.5 hours), and allogeneic blood transfusion.

Postoperative risk factors include woundhealing complications (e.g., superficial infection, hematoma, delayed healing, wound necrosis, and dehiscence), atrial fibrillation, myocardial infarction, urinary tract infection, prolonged hospital stay, and *S. aureus* bacteremia[12-15],[18-21].

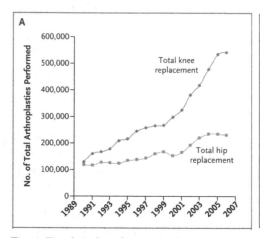 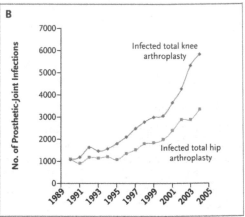

Fig. 1. Total Arthroplasties Performed and Prosthetic Infections, According to Procedure. Panel A shows the number of total arthroplasties performed from 1990 through 2006. Data are from the Centers for Disease Control and Prevention. Panel B shows the number of prosthetic joint infections from 1990 through 2004. Data are from Kurtz et al.

An increased rate of infection occurs in the pre-damaged joint and is also associated with particular predispositions of the patients (Table 1) [22-24]. In articular, a joint prosthesis is a high risk predisposition for an infection. Perioperatively the initial bacterial entry into the joints may occur. On the other hand the implanted foreign material causes in addition to the severe joint disease present an additional reduction in local resistance, which facilitates haematogenous infections. The prosthetic materials are also additional binding sites for various bacteria, and act as a starting point for prosthetic infections. Thus, in addition to the local conditions, the bacterial properties and their specific pathogenity have to be considered for understanding the whole mechanism of infection. Basically, a too late or not

| Preexisting joint defects |
| Extraarticular infection |
| Diabetes mellitus |
| Immunosuppression |
| Higher age |
| Intraarticular injection or operation |
| HLA-B27, for reactive arthritis |

Table 1. Predisposing factors

sufficiently cured joint infection can cause trophic and functional limitations or can even be the starting point of a progressive infection spreading in continuity, lymphogenic or haematogenic. In general, the detection and treatment of acute infectious arthritis is an acute emerging situation, in which a delay may progress to further septic inflammation[23].

3. Classification of the arthroplasty associated infection

The arthroplasty associated infection may distinguishes two major types—septic arthritis and osteomyelitis, which both cause serious morbidity and are often difficult to manage.

Septic arthritis is a joint disease typified by bacterial colonisation and rapid articular destruction[6]. Infiltration and growth of bacteria within the synovium results in inflammation with infiltration of leukocytes into the joint fluid [4]. The production of reactive oxygen species and host matrix metalloproteinases (MMPs), lysosomal enzymes and bacterial toxins contribute to the destruction of cartilage. This starts with degradation of host proteoglycans followed by collagen breakdown within hours of infection, and is mediated by polymorphonuclear leukocytes[3-5,24]. The containment of the inflammatory process within the joint results in increasing pressure, which impedes blood and nutrient supply to the joint exacerbating joint damage and facilitating destruction of cartilage and the synovium. Permanent destruction of articular cartilage and subchondral bone can occur rapidly, within just a few days[24].

Osteomyelitis describes a range of infections in which bone is colonized with microorganisms, with associated inflammation and bone destruction. Acute osteomyelitic foci are characterized by pus-forming inflammation at the site of microbial colonisation. Damage to bone matrix and compression and destruction of vasculature is also observed as the infection spreads to surrounding soft tissues, which can further exacerbate bone necrosis[7,10].Sections of dead bone, known as sequestra, can form which may then detach to form separate infectious foci which, due to the lack of vasculature, are protected from immune cells and antibiotics[7,10]. Such areas of dead, infected tissues that are inaccessible to antimicrobials or the immune response can lead to chronic persistence of the infection[10].

The principal routes of these infection involve: (I) haematogenous or lymphogenous seed of the pathogen, (II) contiguous, by contact with a neighboring infected site, (III) or direct, resulting from infiltration of bone, often following inj ury, surgery or implantation of a foreign body, such as joint repalcement[25]. The range of environments experienced by the bacterium differs for each route and hence the virulence factors that are involved in pathology may be different for each route of infection.

Another classification of arthroplasty associated infection distinguishes acute, chronic and reactive forms, which differ in their type of joint infection and their triggering bacteria.

Infection with virulent organisms (e.g., S. aureus and gram-negative bacilli) inoculated at implantation is typically manifested as acute infection in the first 3 months (or, with hematogenous seeding of the implant, at any time) after surgery, whereas infection with less virulent organisms (e.g., coagulase-negative staphylococci and P. acnes) is more often manifested as chronic infection several months (or years) postoperatively. The most common symptom of infection associated with a prosthetic joint is pain. In acute infection, local signs and symptoms (e.g., severe pain, swelling, erythema, and warmth at the infected joint) and fever are common. Chronic infection generally has a more subtle presentation, with pain alone, and it is often accompanied by loosening of the prosthesis at the bone–cement interface and sometimes by sinus tract formation with discharge.

Reactive arthritis is a postinfectious complication with no need of presence for viable pathogens in the joint. While reactive arthritis often simultaneously affect several joints, the presence of polyarthritic types of non reactive arthritis occur infrequently and then mostly as a result of several bacteriaemic phases.

Among joint infections, the knee is the most frequent localization than others. Infection occurs in 0.8 to 1.9% of knee arthroplasties[12-14]and 0.3 to 1.7% of hip arthroplasties[14-16]. However, hip joint infections are aggravated by the fact that they can exist over a long time with only poor symptoms. Basically, there are no differences in the bacterial spectrum among large joints.

4. Bacteria responsible for arthroplasty associated infection

A broad range of bacterial species have been isolated in cases of septic arthritis and osteomyelitis[26]. Pathogens cultured from septic joints include S. aureus, Streptococcus pyogenes, Streptococcus pneumoniae, Escherichia coli, Pseudomonas aeruginosa, Serratia marcescens, as well as Salmonella, Neisseria, Aerobacter, and Bacteroides species[4,24]. Staphylococcus and Streptococcus spp., Haemophilusinfluenzae, E. coli, P. aeruginosa, Salmonella and Mycobacterium spp. are all potential causes of osteomyelitis[7,10,27].

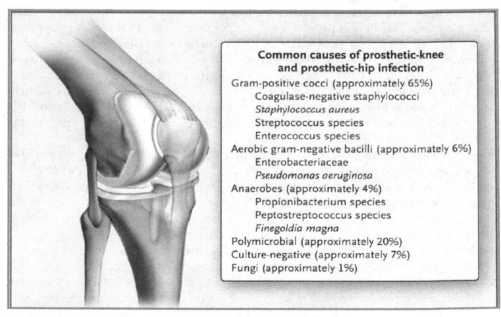

Common causes of prosthetic-knee and prosthetic-hip infection
Gram-positive cocci (approximately 65%)
Coagulase-negative staphylococci
Staphylococcus aureus
Streptococcus species
Enterococcus species
Aerobic gram-negative bacilli (approximately 6%)
Enterobacteriaceae
Pseudomonas aeruginosa
Anaerobes (approximately 4%)
Propionibacterium species
Peptostreptococcus species
Finegoldia magna
Polymicrobial (approximately 20%)
Culture-negative (approximately 7%)
Fungi (approximately 1%)

Fig. 2. Causes of Infection Associated with Prosthetic Joints

A small number of often otherwise nonvirulent bacteria contaminate the implant during surgery and persist as a biofilm despite a functional immune system and antimicrobial treatment. Commonly isolated microorganisms are shown. Unusual organisms that can also cause infection include (but are not limited to) Actinomyces israelii, Aspergillus fumigatus, Histoplasma capsulatum, Sporothrix schenckii, Mycoplasma hominis, Tropheryma whipplei, and mycobacterium (including tuberculosis), brucella, candida, corynebacterium, granulicatella, and abiotrophia species.

Some bacteria have preferences for certain infection routes and patterns. Infections not related to injuries or medical interventions (e.g. intraarticular puncture, joint replacement) are mostly resulting from often physiologic bacteriaemic periods.

S. aureus is the most commonly identified pathogen both in septic arthritis and osteomyelitis, by a substantial margin, regardless of type or route of infection [3,7,28]. Staphylococci (S. aureus and coagulase-negative staphylococcus species) account for more than half of cases of prosthetic-hip and prosthetic-knee infection[29](Fig. 2). Other bacteria

Bacteria	Typical mode of infection
Staphylococci	
Staphylococcus aureus	NJI, PJI
Coagulase negative staphylococci	PJI
Streptococci	
beta-hemolytic (e.g. *Streptococcus pyogenes*)	NJI, RA
Streptococcus pneumoniae	NJI
Enterobacteriaceae	
Escherichia coli	NJI, PJI
Salmonella enterica	
Shigella spec.	
Yersinia spec.	NJI, RAs
Borrelia burgdorferi sensu lato	
Neisseria gonorrhoeae	
Pseudomonas aeruginosa	NJI, PJI
Bartonella henselae	NJI
Mycobacterium tuberculosis and other mycobacteria	
Brucella spp.	NJI
Tropheryma whippelii	
Campylobacter spp.	
Chlamydia trachomatis	RAs
Mycoplasma pneumoniae	
Ureaplasma urealyticum	

Table 2. Bacteria responsible for (hip) joint infections

and fungi cause the remainder of cases[30,31]. Moreover, Staphylococcus aureus has the dominance in acute septic arthritis, and is particularly common in patients with rheumatoid arthritis[32]while coagulase -negative staphylococci can be found mainly in periprosthetic infections and after diagnostic arthroscopies.

Other gram-positive bacteria as causative agents for hip joint infections are streptococci, especially Streptococcus pyogenes, Enterococcus faecalis and Corynebacteria species. Propionibacterium acnes is a common cause of infection associated with shoulder arthroplasty[33].

A large number of different gram-negative rods act as infectious agents on joints. The group of enterobacteria contains a broad spectrum of pathogens. Salmonella enterica, Shigella species, and Yersinia species are classically described as pathogens for purulent and reactive forms of arthritis. Pseudomonas aeruginosa can be found more often in predisposed patients (e.g. diabetics). In otherwise healthy people it is associated with iatrogenic modes of infection during diagnostic procedures.

Campylobacter species, however, are classic agents of reactive arthritis, as well as the obligate intracellular bacteria Chlamydia trachomatis, Mycoplasma pneumoniae, and Ureaplasma urealyticum. From the spirochaetales only Borrelia burgdorferi sensu lato is relevant. Less commonly identified organisms for joint infections often accompanied with osteitis or osteomyelitis are Brucella species and Mycobacterium tuberculosis.

Up to 20% of cases are polymicrobial, most commonly involving methicillin -resistant S. aureus (MRSA) or anaerobes, such as Bacteroides fragilis[34]. Approximately 7% of cases are culture-negative, often in the context of previous antimicrobial therapy[35].

An overview is shown in Table 2[8].

Infection with virulent organisms (e.g., S. aureus and gram-negative bacilli) inoculated at implantation is typically manifested as acute infection in the first 3 months (or, with hematogenous seeding of the implant, at any time) after surgery, whereas infection with less virulent organisms (e.g., coagulase-negative staphylococci and P. acnes) is more often manifested as chronic infection several months (or years) postoperatively.

5. Interaction of staphylococci with bone

5.1 Genomic features of staphylococci associated with bone infections

A number of studies have attempted to identify an association between the possession of certain virulence genes by Staphylococci and invasive disease. Thus Peacock et al.[36]suggested that the possession of certain combinations of virulence factor genes is associated with invasive disease, and increased severity of infection following examination of a panel of 334 S. aureus isolates by PCR. The isolates comprised those from 179 healthy patients, 94 hospitalacquired isolates and 61 community-acquired isolates. Seven putative virulence genes, including the adhesin genes fnbA and cna, the toxin genes sej, eta and hlg, and icaA, which is involved in biofilm production, were found to be associated with invasive isolates. The association with specific types of invasive infection was not examined and indeed the small number of isolates examined in this study would have precluded such an analysis.

The genes for the fibronectin-binding proteins fnbA and fnbB have been reported to be present in 98% and 99% of clinical isolates, respectively, from a range of orthopaedic associated infections, whereas the cna gene, encoding the collagen -binding protein was identified in just 46% of isolates[37]. Another study by Peacock et al.[38]found the prevalence of both fnbA and fnbB genes, as opposed to just one of the two, to be significantly higher in invasive isolates than in 'carriage' strains in a panel of 163 strains, which included septic arthritis and osteomyelitis isolates. Genes encoding Panton-Valentine leukocidin were found to be present in 59 of 89 S. aureus isolates from cases of acute haematogenous osteomyelitis. The presence of pvl genes is associated with an increased risk of severe infection requiring intensive care, bacteremia and more severe systemic inflammation [39,40]. However, one of the problems with the above studies is that it is unclear how representative these strain collections are of those isolates carried in other establishments and regions across the world, since strain typing was not reported.

Strain typing studies of S. aureus, using multilocus sequence typing (MLST) and comparative genomic microarray hybridizations have so far failed to identify any specific clonal lineages associated with invasive disease. However, these studies did not use a collection of isolates from specific invasive diseases and therefore do not rule out the possibility that specific lineages or genes are associated with specific types of infection, such as osteomyelitis or septic arthritis.

To date, the only genome comparison study relevant to S. aureus bone infections has been done using comparative genome microarray hybridisations of the S. aureus UAMS-1 strain, isolated from an osteomyelitis patient, with a range of genome sequenced strains[41]. These authors found variations in the complement of adhesin, toxin, exoenzyme and regulatory genes. Although it is not possible to draw general conclusions about association with bone infection from characterisation of a single strain, the presence of fnbA, but not fnbB or the bone sialoprotein-binding gene bbp, in UAMS-1 suggest that fnbB and bbp are dispensable for bone infection, at least in certain genetic backgrounds. Thus at this juncture there is a lack of evidence to support or disprove an association between specific S. aureus lineages or specific genomic features and the pathogenesis of bone infections.

5.2 Bone as a target organ

In terrestrial vertebrates mature bone is made up of dense surface plates of bone, known as the cortices, and within these is a network of bone struts oriented to oppose loading forces, known as trabecular bone. Trabecular bone is typically replaced every 3-4 years, with the denser cortical bone taking over a decade to replace in adults. This process of continual remodelling is required to remove old bone and microfractures to ensure bone integrity and mineral homeostasis. The skeleton is a dynamic organ system, in a state of perpetual turnover which is continually remodelled by the actions of two cell types, osteoblasts and osteoclasts.

Osteoblasts are responsible for the deposition of bone matrix; they are found on bone surfaces and are derived from mesenchymal steoprogenitor cells. These cells secrete osteoid, a mixture of bone matrix proteins primarily made up of type I collagen (over 90%), proteoglycans such as decorin and biglycan, glycoproteins such as fibronectin, osteonectin and tenascin-C, osteopontin, osteocalcin and bone sialoprotein, oriented along stress lines. Osteoblasts are also thought to facilitate the mineralization of bone matrix, whereby hydroxyapatite, $[Ca_3(PO_4)_2]_3 \cdot Ca[OH]_2$, crystals form, making up around 90% of bone matrix. It is thought that 'nucleators' are required to instigate mineralisation, and phosphate-containing matrix proteins like bone sialoprotein and osteopontin are likely to play such a role. Osteoblasts also produce tissue nonspecific alkaline phosphatase (TNAP) which cleaves phosphate esters to liberate free inorganic phosphate, which is key to the process of mineralisation[42].

Osteoblasts are not terminally differentiated, and some may form osteocytes and become implanted in the bone matrix, eventually ceasing the secretion of osteoid, whilst others undergo apoptosis. Osteocytes are also involved in bone maintenance, detecting stress within the bone through echanosensitive mechanisms located in extensive cellular projections, called canaliculi, that interconnect osteocytes[42]. Osteocytes are thought to respond to mechanical stress by undergoing apoptosis, leading to osteoclast recruitment and differentiation, possibly by alterations in the levels of soluble factors produced by the osteocyte. Candidates include transforming growth factor β (TGF-β), which may suppress osteoclastogenesis when produced by healthy osteocytes[43,44].

Osteoclasts, which are multinucleate cells derived from the acrophage-monocyte lineage, perform the opposing action of bone matrix removal. These cells express large quantities of a vacuolar-type H+-ATPase on their cell surface, along with chloride channel 7 (ClC 7)enabling localised hydrochloric acid secretion into a closed compartment, known as the resorption lacuna, and subsequent olubilisation of bone mineral. The cell is attached to the bone matrix by a sealing zone membrane to create this compartment, and fusion of acidified vesicles with the plasma membrane contributes further to acid release[45].Following mineral solubilisation, proteolysis of bone matrix proteins is then possible. Cathepsin K is centrally involved in degradation of bone matrix, it is highly expressed by osteoclasts and digests substrates such as collagen and osteonectin. Evidence from knock-out mouse and selective inhibitor experiments indicates that cathepsin L, and MMPs also play a role in degrading bone matrix[46]. Osteoclasts also secrete acid phosphatases, such as tartrate-resistant acid phosphatase(TRAcP), which is used as an osteoclast marker and is activated by cathepsin K cleavage. TRAcP is able to generate reactive oxygen species in addition to having phosphatase activity. The exact cellular function of TRAcP in bone resorption is not well understood, but serum TRAcP levels correlate with bone-resorptive activity, and TRAcP-deficient mice exhibit reduced osteoclastic bone resorption and increased bone mineralization.

The balance of activity between these two cell types is crucial to maintaining the proper homeostasis of bone turnover, and any shift in the relative levels of osteoblast and osteoclast activity can result in bone pathology. Infection with a pathogen such as S. aureus is capable of stimulating such a shift, mediated in part by induction of an inflammatory response. There is intimate interaction between the two cell types, with osteoblasts interpreting the majority of extracellular signals and subsequently modulating osteoclast differentiation and function[44].

Interaction between the RANK (receptor activator for nuclear factor κB) receptor, expressed by osteoclast precursors, and its cognate ligand, RANKL, expressed by osteoblasts is essential for osteoclastogenesis [44]. RANKL is a homotrimeric protein displayed on the membrane of osteoblasts, although it may be secreted following cleavage by MMPs 7 or 14, or ADAM (a disintegrin and metalloprotease domain). Suppression of MMP 14-mediated secretion enhances osteoclastogenesis[47,48]. The RANK receptor is a homotrimeric transmembrane protein belonging to the tumour necrosis factor (TNF) receptor superfamily. Following binding of RANKL to RANK, TRAF (TNF receptor-associated factor) adaptor proteins are recruited, with binding sites for TRAF2, TRAF5 and TRAF6 all present on RANK. TRAF6 seems to play a central role in RANK mediated osteoclast formation, and mice deficient in TRAF6 are osteopetrotic whereas TRAF2 and TRAF5 are relatively marginal players in osteoclastogenesis. Signalling via RANK, and these adaptor proteins, activates a number of transcription factors, including NFκB (nuclear factor κB), AP-

1(activator protein 1) and NFATc1 (nuclear factor of activated T-cells, cytoplasmic, calcineurin dependent 1) which drive osteoclast differentiation[44]. Osteoprotegrin (OPG) is an endogenous inhibitor of RANKL signalling, functioning as a decoy receptor that binds to RANKL and prevents its association with RANK.

5.3 Inflammation in bone infection

A number of host cytokines play a significant role in the pathogenesis of osteomyelitis, and there is strong evidence that production of these cytokines is induced by staphylococcal infection of bone, and that they directly contribute to bone destruction. In particular, the inflammatory cytokines tumour necrosis factor α (TNFα), interleukin 1 (IL-1) and IL-6 seem to be especially important in bone physiology and pathology. In patients with acute osteomyelitis, plasma levels of TNFα, IL-1β (the secreted form of IL-1) and IL-6 are all elevated. High levels of IL-1β, IL-6 and TNFα are also found in the synovial fluid of patients with septic arthritis. Interestingly, specific polymorphisms in the IL-1α and IL-6 genes have recently been found to be associated with an increased risk of osteomyelitis in the Greek population[49]. The most recently identified member of the IL-1 cytokine superfamily is IL-33, has been shown to expressed in differentiated osteoblasts and blocks osteoclast formation from bone marrow precursor cells[50].

A number of animal models of S. aureus osteomyelitis reveal that bone infection can lead to elevated levels of these cytokines both locally and systemically. Increased levels of IL-1β have been measured in the tibiae of 22-month-old rats experimentally implanted with S. aureus infected needles, and the same animals have increased circulating levels of IL-6[51]. In a murine osteomyelitis model, bone levels of IL-1β and IL-6 are significantly increased in the early post-infection period, with TNFα rising later during the infection. The local source of these cytokines is not fully clear. Production of IL-1β can be induced in human osteoblast-like cell lines by a variety of stimuli, including TNFα. However, infection of primary mouse osteoblasts with S.aureus results in increased transcription, but not increased protein synthesis or secretion of IL-1β. TNFα is detectable only at low levels in human osteoblasts derived from mesenchymal stem cells and the osteosarcoma cell line MG63.Infiltrating immune cells may therefore be a more likely source of IL-1β and TNFα in bone in response to infection. IL-6 however, is produced by osteoblasts in response to a variety of signals, including infection with S. aureus .

These cytokines have potent effects on the process of bone remodelling, and are strongly implicated in the pathology of osteomyelitis. Cell culture models support the view that IL-1 and TNFα stimulate the proliferation and differentiation of osteoclast progenitors into mature osteoclasts in the presence of osteoblasts. TNFα and IL-1β also stimulate osteoclast-mediated bone resorption, a process which may also require the presence of osteoblasts. Similarly, IL-6 increases bone resorption activity and osteoclast number in cultured mouse calvariae, and stimulates osteoclast differentiation in the presence of osteoblasts. In vivo, local administration of IL-1 and TNF antagonists in a non-human primate model of periodontitis results in significant reduction of osteoclast formation and bone destruction. Intravenous administration of TNFα and IL-1 in mice stimulates bone resorption in a dose-dependent fashion, and deletion of the murine IL-1R, TNF-R1 and TNF-R2 receptors and of caspase-1 significantly decreases osteoclast number and the area of bone resorption in calvariae following lipopolysaccharide (LPS) injection.

IL-1β and TNFα also inhibit the differentiation of mesenchymal stem cells into osteoblast-like cells, and suppress the accompanying mineralisation and increased expression of alkaline phosphatase and procollagen I genes, although only TNFα inhibits osteonectin and osteopontin gene expression[52]. TNFα also decreases production of type I collagen and osteocalcin, and of alkaline phosphatase in a variety of osteoblast cell culture and bone tissue explant models, thereby reducing matrix deposition and mineralisation.

Surface-associated material (SAM) from *S. aureus* stimulates bone resorption and osteoclast formation, and blockade of IL-1 or TNFα signalling completely abolishes this bone resorption activity. Neutralisation of TNFα and IL-6 fully abolishes SAM-stimulated osteoclastogenesis, with antagonism of IL-1 having only a partial effect.

The effect of this SAM on osteoclast formation and stimulation of resorption does not require co-culture with osteoblasts, and does not require RANKL signaling[53]. *S.epidermidis* surface material can also induce bone resorption, by a mechanism that is strongly dependent on TNFα and, to a lesser extent, IL-1.Induction and release of these cytokines in response to pathogen-associated molecules involves two main classes of pattern recognition receptors (PRRs), the Toll-like receptors (TLRs) and NOD-like receptors (NLRs). The production of TNFα and IL-6 by murine macrophages in response to *S. aureus* cell wall preparations is dependent on TLR2, and TLR2-deficient mice exhibit reduced survival of intravenous *S. aureus* infections compared to wild-type counterparts. Signalling through TLRs, in response to microbial ligands such as LPS, 'primes' the cell for IL-1β production by inducing expression of the inactive, pro-form of the cytokine[54,55].IL-1β is synthesised as a 31-kDa precursor molecule, and is processed to produce a 17-kDa active molecule by caspase-1. Caspase-1 activation, and subsequent processing and release of active IL-1β involves assembly of a multiprotein complex known as the inflammasome. This complex consists of caspase-1, the adaptor protein ASC (apoptosis-associated speck-like protein containing a caspase recruitment domain (CARD)) and one of several NLR proteins, of which four are known to associate with inflammasomes[56].Each NLR responds to different activating signals, and although the exact recognition steps remain to be elucidated, reported stimuli include flagellin, anthrax lethal toxin, and muramyl dipeptide. A broad range of stimuli for NLRP3 (NLR family pyrin domain containing 3) have been reported, including *S. aureus*. Although NLRP3 and ASC are essential for IL-1β secretion by murine macrophages in response to *S. aureus*, the stimulating signal is as yet unknown, and deletionof the α-, β- and γ-toxins does not perturb production of the cytokine. The inflammasome is involved in cell death in response to bacterial invasion and although invasion of murine osteoblasts by *S. aureus* induces apoptosis, it is not established whether the inflammasome is involved.

Signalling in response to IL-1 and TNF binding of to their respective receptors leads to eventual activation of the NFκB transcription factor and JNK (c-Jun N-terminal kinase) and p38 MAPK(mitogen-activated protein kinase) signaling[57,58]. Studies with knockout mice have shown that at least one of the p50 or p52 NFκB subunits is required for IL-1-induced osteoclast formation and resorptive activity, indicating that much of the osteoclastogenic activity of IL-1 is dependent on NFκB. TNFα binds to two receptors, TNF type I (TNF-R1) and type II (TNF-R2) receptor which differ in their signaling mechanisms although there is substantial signalling crosstalk between the two receptors. Interestingly, the *S. aureus* virulence factor protein A, in addition to possession of immunoglobulin G-binding activity, is able to bind to the TNF-R1 receptor and stimulates downstream signalling and inflammation.

TNFα mediates the osteoclastogenic activity of RANKL. TNFα production by osteoclast progenitors is induced by RANKL and stimulates osteoclast differentiation in an autocrine manner. Signal transduction involves the activation of Janus family (JAK) tyrosine kinases and subsequent phosphorylation and activation of STAT (signal transducers and activators of transcription) family transcription factors. IL-6 mediates bone resorption indirectly, and has no effect on isolated osteoclasts and IL-6 induction of osteoclastogenesis is dependent on the expression of the IL-6 receptor by osteoblasts, but not osteoclast progenitors.

It is clear that these cytokines have a prominent role in modulating bone turnover, and perturbation of their levels can have profound effects on this process. Although some mechanistic details are currently lacking, there is strong evidence that S. aureus infection of bone initiates local and systemic production of TNFα, IL-1 and IL-6 via host PRRs. Elevated levels of these cytokines then shift the homeostatic balance of bone turnover, increasing osteoclast differentiation and bone resorption and iminishing osteoblast-mediated bone matrix production and mineralisation, thereby driving bone destruction.

5.4 Staphylococcal invasion of bone cells

In addition to staphylococcal induction of inflammatory mediators that modulate the actions of osteoblasts and osteoclasts, bacteria of this genus are involved in more direct interactions with bone cells. Invasion and persistence of S. aureus in 'non-professional phagocytic' host cells in vitro has been described for many different cell types, including epithelial cells, endothelial cells and keratinocytes[59]. In cell culture systems, S. aureus is able to invade cultured osteoblasts from murine, human and embryonic chick sources, and S. epidermidis is also able to invade and grow within cultured osteoblasts. Electron microscopy has demonstrated the presence of bacteria within osteoblasts and osteocytes of embryonic chicks following injection with S. aureus, indicating that internalisation by bone cells also occurs in vivo. Intracellular bacteria inside osteoblasts and osteocytes in a patient with recurrent, long-term osteomyelitis of the fibula have been visualised by light and electron microscopy. More recently Stoodley et al. [60]have demonstrated S. aureus biofilms in an infected total joint arthroplasty. Although not reported in this paper the authors also identified S. aureus within host cells (personal communications, Stoodley). Thus the suggestion that internalisation of S. aureus by bone cells in vivo provides a protective niche for the bacterium, where it is shielded from immune effector mechanisms and antibiotics, may help to explain persistent cases of osteomyelitis. However, the true importance of intracellular staphylococci in clinical osteomyelitis has yet to be established.

S. aureus requires fibronectin-binding proteins (FnBPs) expressed on the surface of the bacterium to enable uptake by osteoblasts, and many other cell types. These proteins belong to a group of adhesions known as MSCRAMMs (microbial surface components recognising adhesive matrix molecules), which bind a range of extracellular matrix proteins including fibronectin, fibrinogen, collagen, elastin and bone sialoprotein. Mutants deficient in the two FnBPs, FnBPA and FnBPB invade host cells very poorly. Invasion is dependent on fibronectin binding by these proteins, and on the host cell integrin $\alpha 5\beta 1$ receptor. S. aureus binds to fibronectin via FnBPs displayed on the bacterial surface, and fibronectin serves as a bridging molecule to the integrin $\alpha 5\beta 1$ which acts as a "phagocytic"receptor. Alternative uptake mechanisms do exist in certain cell types, however, as S. aureus is still able to invade primary keratinocytes in the absence of FnBPs and uptake is not inhibited by blockade of integrin $\alpha 5\beta 1$ binding to fibronectin. The mechanism of invasion also differs between S. aureus and S. epidermidis and the latter does not gain entry via the fibronectin-integrin $\alpha 5\beta 1$ mechanism[61].

The level of expression of the alternative sigma factor, σ B, affects fnbA expression and the fibronectin binding ability of S. aureus strains and correlates with the level of internalization of bacteria by osteoblasts suggesting that σ B-mediated up-regulation of FnBP expression may facilitate invasion[62].

Integrin $\alpha 5 \beta 1$-mediated uptake of S. aureus requires remodelling of the actin cytoskeleton. The integrin-linked kinase, ILK, provides a link between $\alpha 5 \beta 1$ and the cytoskeleton, and interacts with the cytoplasmic domains of β integrins and is subsequently activated. ILK activity is required for internalisation of S. aureus by epithelial cells. Recruitment of focal adhesion proteins, including the adaptor protein paxillin and the focal adhesion kinase, FAK, follows. Upon infection of HEK293T cells with S. aureus there is also recruitment of focal adhesion proteins, such as tensin, zyxin and vinculin to the site of bacterial attachment. FAK is recruited and tyrosine phosphorylated, and FAK-deficient cells are able to internalise S. aureus much less efficiently. Phosphorylation of downstream substrates of FAK, including cortactin, which is involved in actin cytoskeletal organisation, occurs during invasion, and interference with cortactin also reduces internalisation. So, signalling downstream of the integrin $\alpha 5 \beta 1$ receptor, involving ILK and FAK, is important for S. aureus invasion, at least in certain cell types.

Physical contact between S. aureus and osteoblasts induces host cell expression of tumour necrosis factor apoptosis inducing ligand (TRAIL) . TRAIL is a member of the TNF cytokine family, and binds to two death domain -containing receptors, TRAIL receptors 1 and 2, which once activated recruit the FADD (Fas-associated protein with death domain) adaptor protein which in turn activates caspases 8 and −10 and commits the cell to an apoptotic pathway[63]. TRAIL produced by S. aureus-infected osteoblasts induces caspase-8 activation and apoptosis in cultured osteoblasts. Uninfected osteoblasts cultured alongside infected cells also express TRAIL[64]. TRAIL can induce apoptosis in human osteoclasts via TRAIL receptor 2, and also inhibits osteoclast differentiation. It is therefore possible that apoptosis of bone cells infected with S. aureus, and potentially of neighbouring uninfected cells may contribute to bone loss in osteomyelitis .

Growing experimental support indicates that staphylococcal invasion of osteoblasts, most likely via the FnBP-fibronectin-integrin α5β1 bridging mechanism in the case of S. aureus, may play a role in the pathogenesis of bone infections. This intracellular location may provide a protected environment for bacteria, aiding prolonged persistence by enabling evasion of antimicrobials and host immune mechanisms and possibly contributing to bone damage by inducing apoptosis of infected cells.

5.5 Staphylococcal virulence determinants

A number of animal models of bone implant infection, osteomyelitis and septic arthritis have been developed which have enabled the role of specific virulence factors in infections to be determined. As mentioned at the outset there are a number of routes of bone infection, i.e. haematogenous, contiguous and direct infection of bone, and models have been developed to mimic each of these routes of infection. This is important since the range of environments experienced by the bacterium differs for each route and hence the virulence factors that are involved in pathology may be different for each route of infection. The septic arthritis model developed by Tarkowski and colleagues in conjunction with defined isogenic mutants deficient in one or more virulence determinants, or with neutralising antibodies to virulence factors has proven to be particularly useful in elucidating the role of specific virulence determinants and host factors in bone infections. This model has shown that there is a plethora of virulence determinants involved in S. aureus septic arthritis. some of which are also involved in osteomyelitis. However, there is some controversy in this area because whilst the murine septic arthritis model is well established and standardised a number of different models have been developed for osteomyelitis and the relevance of specific virulence factors to bone implant infections or osteomyelitis appears to be dependent on the particular model used. For example the collagen adhesin Cna has been shown to contribute to osteomyelitis by some workers but not by others and has been reported not to be important in orthopaedic device infections. The role of FnBPs has not been directly assessed in a model of osteomyelitis, but comparison of *S. aureus* strains with and without fibronectin-binding activity in a mouse osteomyelitis model suggests that fibronectin-binding strains may give rise to more severe bone infections. In the septic arthritis model, *S. aureus fnbA fnbB* mutants show no reduction in severity of arthritis, in contrast with *clfA clfB* mutants lacking the fibrinogen-binding clumping factors. However, the presence of the *fnb* genes results in greater weight loss and mortality, as well as higher serum levels of IL-6, indicating a role for FnBPs in the systemic inflammatory response.

One area of research that has received surprisingly little attention is that of the direct action of virulence factors on bone and bone cells. Work in our own laboratory has shown that *S.aureus* and *S. epidermidis* produce surface-associated proteins that can stimulate bone breakdown in an in vitro assay. These surface-associated proteins and capsular material appear to promote the formation and activation of the boneresorbing osteoclast. Interestingly, a proportion of the population have antibodies that can block the action of the *S. aureus* proteins and prevent bonebreakdown. The identity of the protein(s) in these mixtures which cause bone destruction has not been elucidated.

5.6 Small colony variants

Variant forms of *S. aureus*, known as small colony variants (SCVs), are associated with infections of bone and joint that may be particularly persistent, recurrent and refractory to antibiotic treatment[65]. These bacteria are mutant forms of *Staphylococcus* that may have an adaptive advantage enabling persistent bone colonisation.

SCV forms of coagulase-negative staphylococci, including *S. epidermidis*, *S. lugdunensis* and *S. capitis* have also been isolated from a range of infections. The SCV phenotype is characterised by slow growth, with colonies around 10-fold smaller than wild-type forms, often with decreased pigmentation, increased aminoglycoside resistance and some reports of reduced haemolytic activity[66]. The nature of these phenotypes can cause difficulty in detection and identification of the bacteria, and may contribute to an underestimation of the clinical prevalence of SCVs [67]. These phenotypes usually result from auxotrophy for hemin, menadione or thymidine and can be reversed by supplementation with these molecules. Mutations in the *hemB* and *menD* genes produce hemin and menadione auxotrophic strains with typical SCV phenotypes, and give rise to disruption of electron transport which is the basis of the growth deficiency, increased minoglycoside resistance and other phenotypes. SCVs can be selected for with gentamicin in vitro, and there is evidence that antibiotic therapy, in particular use of gentamicin beads, which are used in addition to debridement and systemic antibiotic therapy for osteomyelitis may select for SCVs in clinical situations. In a cohort of fourteen patients with confirmed *S. aureus* osteomyelitis, SCVs were isolated only from those four that had received gentamicin bead therapy, with the remaining ten patients harbouring normal *S. aureus* strains. Of the four SCVs, three were auxotrophic for hemin, and one for menadione. Only the patients harbouring SCVs had recurrent infections, although only patients whose gentamicin bead therapy had failed were included in the study. SCVs have also been isolated from cases of infection of hip prostheses, and intracellular bacteria within host fibroblasts were identified in one of the five instances.

Clinically isolated SCVs with hemin auxotrophy, and defined *hemB* mutants, show enhanced intracellular persistence in a range of human cell types. The basis of this persistence is not established but may involve a number of possible mechanisms. *S. aureus* *hemB* mutants exhibit enhanced binding to fibrinogen and fibronectin, and transcribe and display more ClfA and FnBP on their surface, which may increase attachment and uptake by host cells. Transcriptional profiling of clinical and defined mutant SCVs reveals increased transcription of genes regulated by σB, including adhesin genes, and down-regulation of exoprotein and toxin genes. The effect of increased σB activity on MSCRAMM expression has been shown to correlate well with osteoblast invasion, adding weight to the argument that σB-mediated upregulation of adhesins increases host cell invasion, at least in vitro, and that increased invasion by SCVs may be partially dependent on this mechanism. It has been argued that reduced production of toxins, particularly haemolysins, by SCVs also contributes to intracellular persistence by reducing the cytotoxic effect on host cells.

In a murine septic arthritis model, a defined stable *hemB* mutant, exhibiting the SCV phenotype, elicited more frequent and severe arthritis than the parental strain despite a reduced bacterial load in the kidney and joints. It has been argued that SCVs are therefore more virulent on a 'per organism' basis and that enhanced protease production by *hemB* mutants may partially explain this. It may be that in clinical infections relatively small numbers of SCVs with enhanced virulence survive within tissues, possibly intracellularly, for extended periods and cause persistent infections. Clinically isolated SCVs are able to revert to the parent phenotype, although to what extent this may play a role in infections, and whether *S. aureus* may 'switch' between states in different in vivo situations is currently unclear.

6. Diagnostic approach

It is important to accurately diagnose prosthetic-joint–associated infection because its management differs from that of other causes of arthroplasty failure. Although there is no universally accepted definition of this type of infection, the criteria listed in Table 3 have been applied in a number of studies.

The presence of at least one of the following findings:
• Acute inflammation detected on histopathological examination of periprosthetic tissue
• Sinus tract communicating with the prosthesis
• Gross purulence in the joint space
• Isolation of the same microorganism from two or more cultures of joint aspirates or intraoperative periprosthetic-tissue specimens, isolation of the organism in substantial amounts (e.g., ≥20 CFU per 10 ml from the implant in a total volume of 400 ml of sonicate fluid), or both

Table 3. Criteria for the Diagnosis of a Prosthetic-Joint Infection.

Establishing the presence of acute infection or, in the presence of a draining sinus, chronic infection, is uncomplicated. In these situations, testing may be limited to that needed to establish the microbiologic diagnosis. Chronic infection manifested as localized joint pain alone poses more diagnostic difficulty, warranting additional testing. The criteria for interpreting laboratory and imaging findings in patients with a prosthetic joint are distinct from those applied in patients with a native joint. In addition to establishing the diagnosis, the identification of the involved organism or organisms and their antimicrobial susceptibility (i.e., on the basis of cultures of synovial fluid, periprosthetic tissue, the implant, or a combination of such cultures) is important in order to guide antimicrobial therapy.

C-Reactive Protein—In the absence of underlying inflammatory conditions, CRP measurement is the most useful preoperative blood test for detecting infection associated with a prosthetic joint. CRP testing has a sensitivity of 73 to 91% and a specificity of 81 to 86% for the diagnosis of prosthetic-knee infection with the use of a cutoff point of 13.5 mg per liter or more[68,69]. It has a sensitivity of 95% and a specificity of 62% for the diagnosis of prosthetichip infection with the use of a cutoff point of more than 5 mg per liter[70]. Although the CRP level and erythrocyte sedimentation rate are elevated after uncomplicated arthroplasty, the CRP level returns to the preoperative level within 2 months, whereas the erythrocyte edimentation rate may remain elevated for several months. A normal CRP level generally indicates an absence of infection, although false negative results may occur in patients who have been treated with antimicrobial agents or who have infection that is caused by low-virulenceorganisms such as *P. acnes*. Elevations in the peripheral -blood leukocyte count and levels of procalcitonin have low sensitivity for detecting infection.

Imaging—Plain radiography has low sensitivity and low specificity for detecting infection associated with a prosthetic joint[71]. Periprosthetic radiolucency, osteolysis, migration, or all of these features may be present on radiographs in patients with either infection or aseptic loosening of the prosthesis. Diagnostic studies with the use of computed tomography (CT) or magnetic resonance imaging (MRI) are hampered by artifacts produced by prostheses, although implants that are not ferromagnetic (i.e., titanium or tantalum) are associated with minimal MRI artifacts, and MRI scans of such implants provide good resolution for detecting soft-tissue abnormalities. Bone scans obtained after the administration of technetium-99m –labeled methylene diphosphonate are sensitive for detecting failed implants but nonspecific for detecting infection, and they may remain abnormal for more than a year after implantation.

Some studies suggest that combined bone and gallium-67 scans are more specific than bone scans alone. However, labeled-leukocyte imaging (e.g., leukocytes labeled with indium-111) combined with bone marrow imaging with the use of technetium -99m–labeled sulfur colloid is more accurate than bone imaging alone, combined bone and gallium-67 imaging, or labeledleukocyte and bone imaging when compared head to head, and it is considered the imaging test of choice when imaging is required[71]. 18F-fluorodeoxyglucose positron-emission tomography (PET) has a sensitivity of 82% and a specificity of 87% for the detection of prosthetic-knee or prosthetic-hip infection, on the basis of pooled data from several studies, but it is not widely available[72]. Newer imaging strategies such as scintigraphy with antigranulocyte monoclonal antibodies and hybrid imaging (e.g., combined PET and CT) (see Fig. 3)are under investigation.

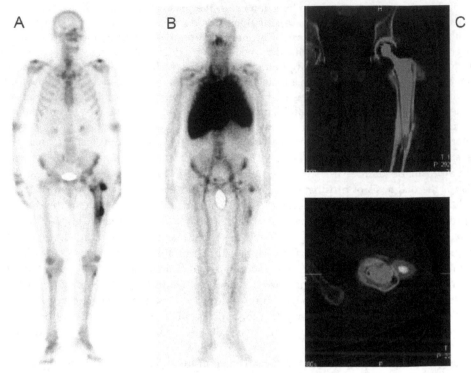

Fig. 3. Bone Scan, Labeled-Leukocyte Scan and Positron Emission Tomography/Computed Tomography Scan from a Patient with Prosthetic Joint Infection.

In Panel A, an anterior bone scan obtained after the administration of technetium-99m–labeled methylene diphosphonate shows diffusely increased activity around the femoral component of a left hip replacement, with foci of increased activity at the tip of the femoral component and around the tibia. In Panel B, a labeled leukocyte scan obtained after the administration of indium-111–labeled leukocytes shows accumulation of labeled leukocytes that is spatially congruent with the bone scan image shown in Panel A. In Panel C, 18F-fluoro-2-deoxyglucose positron emission tomography/computed tomography coronal and sagittal images show increased activity around the bone-prosthesis interface. Staphylococcus epidermidis and Finegoldia magna were isolated from the periprosthetic tissue. (Images courtesy of Carmen Vigil, M.D., and Jose Angel Richter, M.D., Department of Nuclear Medicine, University Hospital of Navarre, Pamplona, Spain.)

Synovial-Fluid Studies—If there is uncertainty about the diagnosis, the most useful preoperative diagnostic test is aspiration of joint synovial fluid for a total and differential cell count and culture. Aspiration should not be performed through overlying cellulitis. Hip aspiration may require imaging guidance. A synovial-fluid leukocyte count of more than $1.7×10^3$ per cubic millimeter or a differential count with more than 65% neutrophils is consistent with prosthetic-knee infection. A synovial-fluid leukocyte count of more than $4.2×10^3$ per cubic millimeter or more than 80% neutrophils is consistent with prosthetic-hip infection[73]. The leukocyte count cutoffs are dramatically lower than those used to diagnose native-joint infection. Synovial-fluid culture has a sensitivity of 56 to 75% and a specificity of 95 to 100%, and to achieve optimal sensitivity and specificity, it should be performed by means of inoculation into a blood-culture bottle. If an organism of questionable clinical significance is isolated, repeat synovial-fluid aspiration for culture should be considered. Previous antimicrobial treatment reduces the sensitivity.

Histopathological Examination of Periprosthetic Tissue — In patients in whom the diagnosis of prosthetic-joint–associated infection has not been established preoperatively, an intraoperative frozen section may be obtained to look for evidence of acute inflammation. In studies that used a polymorphonuclear-cell count ranging from more than 5 to 10 or more cells per high-power field as a positive test, sensitivity for infection ranged from 50 to 93% and specificity ranged from 77 to 100%; the rate of interobserver agreement was 86%.

Intraoperative Microbiologic Testing — Identification of the pathogen or pathogens is critical for choosing the antimicrobial regimen; if microbiologic testing has not been done preoperatively, specimens should be collected for microbiologic study at the time of surgery. Antimicrobial therapy should be discontinued at least 2 weeks before surgery, and perioperative antimicrobial coverage should be deferred until culture specimens have been collected. Cultures of sinus tract exudates should be avoided; these are often positive because of microbial skin colonization and correlate poorly with cultures of surgical specimens.

If periprosthetic tissue is obtained, collection of multiple periprosthetic-tissue specimens for aerobic and anaerobic bacterial culture is imperative because of the poor sensitivity of a single culture and to distinguish contaminants from pathogens. A study that used mathematical modeling to estimate yield based on the number of cultures concluded that to maximize accuracy, five or six specimens should be submitted for culture, and two or three culturepositive samples would be considered to be diagnostic.

Periprosthetic-tissue cultures may be falsely negative because of previous antimicrobial therapy, leaching of antimicrobial agents from antimicrobial -impregnated cement, biofilm growth on the surface of the prosthesis (but not in the surrounding tissue), a low number of organisms in tissue, an inappropriate culture medium, an inadequate culture incubation time, or a prolonged time to transport the specimen to the laboratory. Because of poor sensitivity, neither intraoperative swab cultures nor Gram's staining of the periprosthetic tissue is recommended. Fungal cultures, mycobacterial cultures, or both may be considered (e.g., if bacterial cultures are negative in a patient with apparent infection), but they are not routinely recommended.

Microorganisms form a biofilm on the prosthesis; therefore, if the prosthesis is removed, obtaining a sample from its surface is useful for microbiologic diagnosis. The implant is removed and transported to the laboratory in a sterile jar. After the addition of Ringer's solution, the container is vortexed and sonicated (frequency, 40 kHz; power density, 0.22 W per square centimeter) for 5 minutes in a bath sonicator, and the resultant fluid is cultured. This technique is more sensitive than and as specific as multiple periprosthetic-tissue cultures for diagnosing infection of a prosthetic hip, knee, or shoulder, provided that an appropriate cutoff for significant results is applied. This technique is particularly helpful in patients who have received previous antimicrobial therapy. In a study involving patients receiving antimicrobial agents within 2 weeks before surgery, the sensitivity of periprosthetic-tissue culture was 45%, whereas the sensitivity of sonicate-fluid culture was 75% (P<0.001). Sonication in bags is not recommended because of the potential for contamination.

6.1 Treatment

The goal of treatment is to cure the infection, prevent its recurrence, and ensure a pain-free, functional joint. This goal can best be achieved by a multidisciplinary team consisting of an orthopedic surgeon, an infectious-disease specialist, and a clinical microbiologist. On the basis of clinical experience, the use of antimicrobial agents alone, without surgical intervention, ultimately fails in most cases. Careful surgical débridement is critical. A general approach to surgical management is outlined in Figure 4; different centers and surgeons may use slightly different strategies. Chronic infections require resection arthroplasty either as a onstage exchange (i.e., removal of the infected prosthesis and reimplantation of a new prosthesis during the same surgical procedure) or a two-stage exchange (i.e., removal of the infected prosthesis and administration of systemic antimicrobial agents with subsequent implantation of a new prosthesis, usually between 6 weeks and 3 months after the first stage). Case series have suggested improved outcomes with a one-stage exchange when polymethylmethacrylate impregnated with one or more antimicrobial agents is used. A spacer impregnated with one or more antimicrobial agents may be used to maintain the leg at its correct length and to control infection during the prosthesis-free interval of a two-stage exchange. In a randomized trial involving patients with infection associated with hip arthroplasty, the use of a vancomycinloaded spacer (as compared with no spacer) resulted in a lower rate of recurrent infection (11% vs. 33%, P = 0.002)[74].

Patients who have had symptoms of infection for fewer than 3 weeks, who present with infection within 3 months after implantation or who have hematogenous infection, and who have a well-fixed, functioning prosthesis, without a sinus tract, and with an appropriate microbiologic diagnosis (Fig. 4) may be candidates for débridement and retention of the prosthesis. The addition of rifampin is recommended in cases of rifampin-susceptible staphylococcal infection. In a small, randomized trial comparing different antibiotic regimens in patients with staphylococcal infection of prosthetic knees or hips or osteosynthetic implants, salvage of the implant was successful in all 12 patients treated for 3 to 6 months with rifampin and ciprofloxacin, as compared with successful salvage in 7 of 12 patients treated with ciprofloxacin alone for 3 to 6 months (P = 0.02).

When unacceptable joint function is anticipated after surgery or the infection has been refractory to multiple surgical attempts at cure, resection arthroplasty with creation of a pseudarthrosis for hips (Girdlestone resection) or arthrodesis for knees may be considered. If the patient is not a candidate for surgery, antimicrobial suppression may be attempted; this approach is unlikely to cure infection, so the use of antimicrobial agents is often continued indefinitely.

In brief, information about antimicrobial susceptibility should be used to confirm the activity of any antimicrobial agent used for therapy. Data from randomized trials on the optimal duration of treatment are lacking. The therapeutic approach has to be selected in accordance with the mode of infection (NJI, PJI, RA), the expected or found pathogens, and their resistance. It should be remembered that the slowed growth of bacteria in a biofilm on surfaces of joint prosthesis may additionally reinforces antibiotic resistance. Responsible for such an increase against antibacterial substances are changes in cell wall synthesis, which limits the effect of beta-lactam antibiotics and glycopeptides, and the occurrence of bacterial variants with modifications of other metabolic activities, with implications for the action of quinolones, aminoglycosides, and tetracyclines. In principle, the spectrum of available antibiotics is limited by the specific pharmacokinetic requirements in the treatment of joint infections. This applies particularly to chronic infections and prosthesis infections.

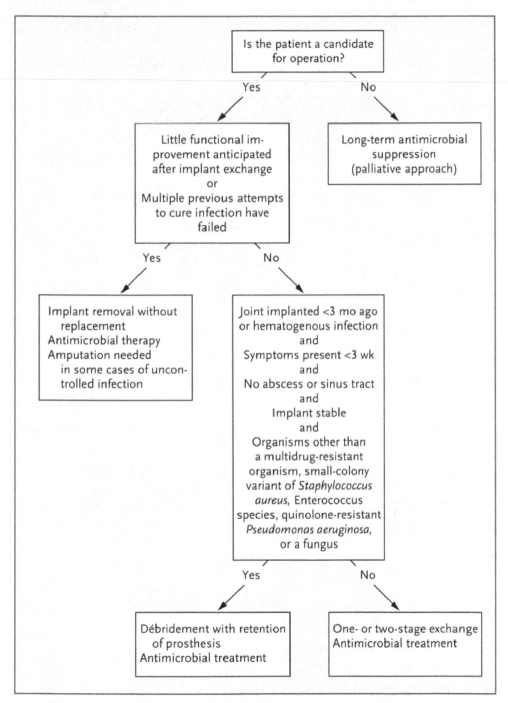

Fig. 4. Algorithm for the Treatment of Infection Associated with a Prosthetic joint

Organism	Antibiotics	
	Native joint infection	Prosthetic joint infection
Methicillin resistant *Staphylococcus aureus*	(I) First choice: Vancomycin 2× 1 g/d Linezolid 2× 600 mg/d (II) Alternatives: Cotrimoxazol, Doxycyclin, Clindamycin, Rifampicin (always in combination)	(I) First choice (in combination with Rifampicin 600–900 mg): Vancomycin 2× 1 g/d Teicoplanin 800 mg/d for the first 1–4 days, than 800 mg every 2 days Fluoroquinolone (e.g. Ciprofloxacin 2× 500–750 mg/d) Fusidinsäure 3× 500 mg/d (II) Alternatives: Linezolid, Quinupristin/Dalfopristin
Methicillin resistant coagulase negative staphylococci		
Methicillin sensitive *Staphylococcus aureus*	(I) First choice: beta-lactamase stable penicillin (e.g. Flucloxacillin 4× 2–3 g/d, Nafcillin 4× 2 g/d) Clindamycin 3× 600–900 mg/d (II) Alternatives: Cefazolin, Vancomycin	(I) First choice (in combination with Rifampicin 600–900 mg): Flucloxacillin 4× 2–3 g/d Fluoroquinolone (e.g. Ciprofloxacin 2× 500–750 mg/d) (II) Alternatives (in combination with Rifampicin): Cefazolin, Vancomycin
Methicillin sensitive coagulase negative staphylococci		
beta-hemolytic Streptococci	(I) First choice: Penicillin G 6× 2 million units/d Ampicillin 3× 2 g/d (II) Alternatives: Clindamycin, Cefazolin	(I) First choice Penicillin G 6× 4–5 million units/d Ampicillin 3× 4 g/d (II) Alternatives: Vancomycin, Ceftriaxon
Enterococcus spec.	(I) First choice: Ampicillin 3× 2 g/d Vancomycin 2× 1 g /d (II) Alternatives: Linezolid	(I) First choice Ampicillin 3× 4 g/d Vancomycin 2× 1 g /d Teicoplanin 800 mg/d for the first 1–4 days, than 800 mg every 2 days (II) Alternatives: Linezolid
Escherichia coli	(I) First choice: Ampicillin/Sulbactam 4× 3 g/d (II) Alternatives: Cefazolin, Fluoroquinolone (e.g. Ciprofloxacin), Gentamicin, Cotrimoxazole	
Proteus mirabilis	(I) First choice: Ampicillin 3× 2 g/d Fluoroquinolone (e.g. Ciprofloxacin 2× 500–750 mg/d) (II) Alternatives: Cefazolin, Cotrimoxazole, Gentamicin	(I) First choice: Ciprofloxacin 2× 500–750 mg/d Cefotaxime 3–4× 2 g/d Piperacillin/Tazobactam 3× 4 g/0,5g/d (II) Alternatives: Imipenem, Meropenem
Proteus vulgaris Proteus rettgeri Morganella morganii	(I) First choice: Cefotaxime 3–4× 2 g/d Imipenem 4× 500 mg/d Fluoroquinolone (e.g. Ciprofloxacin 2× 500–750 mg/d) (II) Alternatives: Ampicillin, Gentamicin, free or fixed combination of beta-lactam/beta-lactamase inhibitor (e.g. combinations with Combactam or as Ampicillin/Sulbactam, Piperacillin/Tazobactam, Ticarcillin/Clavulanate)	
Serratia marcescens	(I) First choice: Cefotaxime 3–4× 2 g/d (II) Alternatives: Fluoroquinolone (e.g. Ciprofloxacin) Gentamicin, Imipenem	I) First choice: Ceftazidim 3× 2 g/d + Fluoroquinolone (e.g. Ciprofloxacin 2× 500–750 mg/d) (II) Alternatives: Imipenem, Meropenem
Pseudomonas aeruginosa	(I) First choice: Piperacillin 4× 3 g/d Imipenem 4× 500 mg/d (II) Alternatives: Fluoroquinolone (e.g. Ciprofloxacin) Tobramycin, Amikacin	
Anaerobe infection	(I) First choice: Clindamycin 3× 600–900 mg/d Imipenem 4× 500 mg/d Metronidazole 3× 500 mg/d (II) Alternatives: free or fixed combination of beta-lactam/beta-lactamase inhibitor (e.g. combinations with Combactam or as Ampicillin/Sulbactam, Piperacillin/Tazobactam, Ticarcillin/Clavulanate)	First choice: Clindamycin 3× 600–900 mg/d Piperacillin/Tazobactam 3× 4 g/0,5g/d Imipenem 4× 500 mg/d

(all given dosages are for healthy adults of 70 kg with normal liver and kidney function)

Table 4. Antibiotics for therapy of infectious arthritis

Lysostaphin is a 27 kDa endopeptidase that was first isolated from a culture of Staphylococcus simulans by Schindler & Schuhardt. The enzyme kills the organism by hydrolysing a pentaglycine cross-bridge structure unique to the staphylococcal cell wall. As the cell wall cross-bridges of S. aureus are composed of a high proportion of pentaglycine, both proliferating and quiescent S. aureus cells are highly sensitive to lysostaphin. Lysostaphin kills meticillin-susceptible S. aureus (MSSA) and MRSA equally well and has been demonstrated to be a potent therapeutic agent for S. aureus infections in various animal studies. In the USA, two therapeutic products formulated with recombinant lysostaphin for topical use have entered clinical studies. And recombinant lysostaphin is expected to be a potential alternative therapy for S. aureus infection[78].

For an overview of common substances and therapeutic regimes, see Table 4.

In patients undergoing débridement with retention of the prosthesis, 3-month courses of treatment for infection associated with hip prostheses and 6-month courses for infection associated with knee prostheses are often used. Oral therapy can be used if the agent has good oral bioavailability (e.g., quinolones, rimethoprim– sulfamethoxazole, and tetracyclines). In patients undergoing a two-stage exchange, systemic antimicrobial therapy is often administered for 4 to 6 weeks. Commercially available, preblended, polymethylmethacrylate impregnated with an antimicrobial agent is indicated for use in the second stage of a two-stage revision after elimination of active infection. Although it is not standard clinical practice, two studies involving a long period between the initial and second stages suggest that when a polymethylmethacrylate spacer impregnated with one or more antimicrobial agents or impregnated beads are used, the administration of systemic antimicrobial therapy for 2 weeks may be sufficient or systemic therapy may even be unnecessary[75,76].

6.2 Prophylaxis

In addition to good aseptic technique and procedures in the operating room, the administration of intravenous antimicrobial agents immediately before surgery minimizes the risk of infection. Cefazolin at a dose of 1 g (2 g if the patient weighs ≥ 80 kg) every 8 hours or cefuroxime at a dose of 1.5 g, followed by 750 mg every 8 hours is recommended routinely; vancomycin at a dose of 15 mg per kilogram every 12 hours (assuming normal renal function) is used in patients with a β-lactam allergy or MRSA colonization. Prophylaxis should begin within 60 minutes before surgical incision (within 120 minutes if vancomycin is used) and should be completed within 24 hours after the end of surgery. The entire antimicrobial dose should be infused before inflation of a tourniquet[77].

7. References

[1] National Hospital Discharge Survey: survey results and products. Atlanta: Centers for Disease Control and Prevention; 2009 [Accessed July 24, 2009].
http://www.cdc.gov/nchs/nhds/nhds_products.htm

[2] Lee K. Goodman S.B. Current state and future of joint replacements in the hip and knee. Expert Rev. Med. Devices 2008;5:383–393. [PubMed: 18452388]

[3] Goldenberg D.L. Septic arthritis. Lancet 1998;351:197-202. [PubMed: 9449882]

[4] Nade S. Septic arthritis. Best. Pract. Res. Clin. Rheumatol. 2003;17:183-200. [PubMed: 12787520]

[5] Stott N.S. Paediatric bone and joint infection. J. Orthop. Surg. (Hong Kong) 2001;9:83-90. [PubMed: 12468850]

[6] Levine M. Siegel L.B. A swollen joint: why all the fuss? Am. J. Ther. 2003;10:219–224. [PubMed: 12756429]

[7] Lew D.P. Waldvogel F.A. Osteomyelitis. Lancet 2004;364:369–379. [PubMed: 15276398]

[8] Weichert S. Sharland M. Clarke N.M. Faust S.N. Acute haematogenous osteomyelitis in children: is there any evidence for how long we should treat? Curr. Opin. Infect. Dis. 2008;21:258–262. [PubMed: 18448970]

[9] Blyth M.J. Kincaid R. Craigen M.A. Bennet G.C. The changing epidemiology of acute and subacute haematogenous osteomyelitis in children. J. Bone Joint Surg. Br. 2001;83:99–102. [PubMed: 11245548]

[10] Lazzarini L. Mader J.T. Calhoun J.H. Osteomyelitis in long bones. J. Bone Joint Surg. Am. 2004;86-A: 2305–2318. [PubMed: 15466746]

[11] Gillespie W.J. Epidemiology in bone and joint infection. Infect. Dis. Clin. North Am. 1990;4:361–376. [PubMed: 2212594]

[12] Jämsen E, Huhtala H, Puolakka T, Moilanen T. Risk factors for infection after knee arthroplasty: a register-based analysis of 43,149 cases. J Bone Joint Surg Am 2009;91:38–47.

[13] Peersman G, Laskin R, Davis J, Peterson M. Infection in total knee replacement: a retrospective review of 6489 total knee replacements. Clin Orthop Relat Res 2001;392:15–23. [PubMed: 11716377]

[14] Pulido L, Ghanem E, Joshi A, Purtill JJ, Parvizi J. Periprosthetic joint infection: the incidence, timing, and predisposing factors. Clin Orthop Relat Res 2008;466:1710–5. [PubMed: 18421542]

[15] Choong PF, Dowsey MM, Carr D, Daffy J, Stanley P. Risk factors associated with acute hip prosthetic joint infections and outcome of treatment with a rifampin-based regimen. Acta Orthop 2007;78:755– 65. [PubMed: 18236181]

[16] Phillips JE, Crane TP, Noy M, Elliott TS, Grimer RJ. The incidence of deep prosthetic infections in a specialist orthopaedic hospital: a 15-year prospective survey. J Bone Joint Surg Br 2006;88:943–8. [PubMed: 16799001]

[17] Kurtz SM, Lau E, Schmier J, Ong KL, Zhao K, Parvizi J. Infection burden for hip and knee arthroplasty in the United States. J Arthroplasty 2008;23:984–91. [PubMed: 18534466]

[18] Murdoch DR, Roberts SA, Fowler VG Jr, et al. Infection of orthopedic prostheses after *Staphylococcus aureus bacteremia*. Clin Infect Dis 2001;32:647–9. [PubMed: 11181131]

[19] Berbari EF, Hanssen AD, Duffy MC, et al. Risk factors for prosthetic joint infection: case-control study. Clin Infect Dis 1998;27:1247–54. [PubMed: 9827278]

[20] Bongartz T, Halligan CS, Osmon DR, et al. Incidence and risk factors of prosthetic joint infection after total hip or knee replacement in patients with rheumatoid arthritis. Arthritis Rheum 2008;59:1713–20. [PubMed: 19035425]

[21] Dowsey MM, Choong PF. Obesity is a major risk factor for prosthetic infection after primary hip arthroplasty. Clin Orthop Relat Res 2008;466:153–8. [PubMed: 18196388]

[22] Kaandorp CJ, Krijnen P, Moens HJ, Habbema JD, van Schaardenburg D. The outcome of bacterial arthritis: a prospective community-based study. Arthritis Rheum. 1997; 40:884–92.

[23] Kaandorp CJ, van Schaardenburg D, Krijnen P, Habbema JD, van de Laar MA. Risk factors for septic arthritis in patients with joint disease. A prospective study. Arthritis Rheum. 1995; 38:1819-25.

[24] Shirtliff ME, Mader JT. Acute septic arthritis. Clin Microbiol Rev. 2002; 15: 527-44.

[25] Udo Geipel. Pathogenic organisms in hip joint infections. International Journal of Medical Sciences 2009; 6(5):234-240.

[26] Jose L. Del Pozo, M.D., Ph.D. and Robin Patel, M.D. Infection Associated with Prosthetic Joints. N Engl J Med. 2009 August 20; 361(8): 787-794.

[27] Bennet G.C. Bennet S.J. Infection of bone and joint. Surgery (Oxford) 2006;24:211-214.

[28] Ciampolini J. Harding K.G. Pathophysiology of chronic bacterial osteomyelitis. Why do antibiotics fail so often? Postgrad. Med. J. 2000;76:479-483. [PubMed: 10908375]

[29] Trampuz A, Piper KE, Jacobson MJ, et al. Sonication of removed hip and knee prostheses for diagnosis of infection. N Engl J Med 2007;357:654-63. [PubMed: 17699815]

[30] Marculescu CE, Berbari EF, Cockerill FR III, Osmon DR. Fungi, mycobacteria, zoonotic and other organisms in prosthetic joint infection. Clin Orthop Relat Res 2006;451:64-72. [PubMed: 16906078]

[31] Unusual aerobic and anaerobic bacteria associated with prosthetic joint infections. Clin Orthop Relat Res 2006;451:55-63. Idem. [PubMed: 16906072]

[32] Berbari EF, Osmon DR, Duffy MC, et al. Outcome of prosthetic joint infection in patients with rheumatoid arthritis: the impact of medical and surgical therapy in 200 episodes. Clin Infect Dis 2006;42:216-23. [PubMed: 16355332]

[33] Piper KE, Jacobson MJ, Cofield RH, et al. Microbiologic diagnosis of prosthetic shoulder infection by use of implant sonication. J Clin Microbiol 2009;47:1878-84. [PubMed: 19261785]

[34] Marculescu CE, Cantey JR. Polymicrobial prosthetic joint infections: risk factors and outcome. Clin Orthop Relat Res 2008;466:1397-404. [PubMed: 18421538]

[35] Berbari EF, Marculescu C, Sia I, et al. Culture-negative prosthetic joint infection. Clin Infect Dis 2007;45:1113-9. [PubMed: 17918072]

[36] Peacock S.J. Moore C.E. Justice A. Kantzanou M. Story L. Mackie K. O'Neill G. Day N.P. Virulent combinations of adhesin and toxin genes in natural populations of Staphylococcus aureus. Infect. Immun. 2002;70:4987-4996. [PubMed: 12183545]

[37] Arciola C.R. Campoccia D. Gamberini S. Baldassarri L. Montanaro L. Prevalence of cna, fnbA and fnbB adhesin genes among Staphylococcus aureus isolates from orthopedic infections associated to different types of implant. FEMS Microbiol. Lett. 2005;246:81-86. [PubMed: 15869965]

[38] Peacock S.J. Day N.P. Thomas M.G. Berendt A.R. Foster T.J. Clinical isolates of Staphylococcus aureus exhibit diversity in fnb genes and adhesion to human fibronectin. J. Infect. 2000;41:23-31. [PubMed: 10942636]

[39] Bocchini C.E. Hulten K.G. Mason E.O. Gonzalez B.E. Hammerman W.A. Kaplan S.L. Panton-Valentine leukocidin genes are associated with enhanced inflammatory response and local disease in acute hematogenous Staphylococcus aureus osteomyelitis in children. Pediatrics 2006;117:433-440. [PubMed: 16452363]

[40] Sdougkos G. Chini V. Papanastasiou D.A. Christodoulou G. Tagaris G. Dimitracopoulos G. Spiliopoulou I. Methicillin-resistant Staphylococcus aureus

producing Panton-Valentine leukocidin as a cause of acute osteomyelitis in children. Clin. Microbiol. Infect. 2007;13:651–654. [PubMed: 17371535]

[41] Cassat J.E. Dunman P.M. McAleese F. Murphy E. Projan S.J. Smeltzer M.S. Comparative genomics of Staphylococcus aureus musculoskeletal isolates. J. Bacteriol. 2005;187:576–592. [PubMed: 15629929]

[42] van de Lest C.H. Vaandrager A.B. Mechanism of cell-mediated mineralization. Curr. Opin. Orthop. 2007;18:434–443.

[43] Henriksen K. Neutzsky-Wulff A.V. Bonewald L.F. Karsdal M.A. Local communication on and within bone controls bone remodeling. Bone 2009;44:1026–1033. [PubMed: 19345750]

[44] Matsuo K. Irie N. Osteoclast-osteoblast communication. Arch. Biochem. Biophys. 2008;473:201–209. [PubMed: 18406338]

[45] Vaananen H.K. Laitala-Leinonen T. Osteoclast lineage and function. Arch. Biochem. Biophys. 2008;473:132–138. [PubMed: 18424258]

[46] Everts V. Korper W. Hoeben K.A. Jansen I.D. Bromme D. Cleutjens K.B. Heeneman S. Peters C. Reinheckel T. Saftig P. Beertsen W. Osteoclastic bone degradation and the role of different cysteine proteinases and matrix metalloproteinases: differences between calvaria and long bone. J. Bone Miner. Res. 2006;21:1399–1408. [PubMed: 16939398]

[47] Boyce B.F. Xing L. Functions of RANKL/RANK/OPG in bone modeling and remodeling. Arch. Biochem. Biophys. 2008;473:139–146. [PubMed: 18395508]

[48] Hikita A. Yana I. Wakeyama H. Nakamura M. Kadono Y. Oshima Y. Nakamura K. Seiki M. Tanaka S. Negative regulation of osteoclastogenesis by ectodomain shedding of receptor activator of NfkappaB ligand. J. Biol. Chem. 2006;281:36846–36855. [PubMed: 17018528]

[49] Tsezou A. Poultsides L. Kostopoulou F. Zintzaras E. Satra M. Kitsiou-Tzeli S. Malizos K.N. Influence of interleukin 1alpha (IL-1alpha), IL-4, and IL-6 polymorphisms on genetic susceptibility to chronic osteomyelitis. Clin. Vaccine Immunol. 2008;15:1888–1890. [PubMed: 18971305]

[50] Jochen Schulze.Thomas Bickert.F. Timo Beil.et al. Interleukin-33 is Expressed in Differentiated Osteoblasts and Blocks Osteoclast Formation from Bone Marrow Precursor Cells. Journal of Bone and Mineral Research.

[51] Garcia-Alvarez F. Navarro-Zorraquino M. Castro A. Grasa J.M. Pastor C. Monzon M. Martinez A. Garcia-Alvarez I. Castillo J. Lozano R. Effect of age on cytokine response in an experimental model of osteomyelitis. Biogerontology 2009;10:649–658. [PubMed: 19123052]

[52] Lacey D.C. Simmons P.J. Graves S.E. Hamilton J.A. Proinflammatory cytokines inhibit osteogenic differentiation from stem cells: implications for bone repair during inflammation. Osteoarthritis Cartilage 2008;17:735–742. [PubMed: 19136283]

[53] Lau Y.S. Wang W. Sabokbar A. Simpson H. Nair S. Henderson B. Berendt A. Athanasou N.A. Staphylococcus aureus capsular material promotes osteoclast formation. Injury 2006;37(Suppl. 2):S41–S48. [PubMed: 16651071]

[54] Creagh E.M. O'Neill L.A. TLRs, NLRs and RLRs: a trinity of pathogen sensors that co-operate in innate immunity. Trends Immunol. 2006;27:352–357. [PubMed: 16807108]

[55] Kahlenberg J.M. Lundberg K.C. Kertesy S.B. Qu Y. Dubyak G.R. Potentiation of caspase-1 activation by the P2×7 receptor is dependent on TLR signals and requires NF-kappaB-driven protein synthesis. J. Immunol. 2005;175:7611–7622. [PubMed: 16301671]

[56] Ting J.P.Y. Willingham S.B. Bergstralh D.T. NLRs at the intersection of cell death and immunity. Nat. Rev. Immunol. 2008;8:372–379. [PubMed: 18362948]

[57] Arend W.P. Palmer G. Gabay C. IL-1, IL-18, and IL-33 families of cytokines. Immunol. Rev. 2008;223:20–38. [PubMed: 18613828]

[58] Dinarello C.A. Immunological and inflammatory functions of the interleukin-1 family. Annu. Rev. Immunol. 2009;27:519–550. [PubMed: 19302047]

[59] Garzoni C. Kelley W.L. Staphylococcus aureus: new evidence for intracellular persistence. Trends Microbiol. 2009;17:59–65. [PubMed: 19208480]

[60] Stoodley P. Nistico L. Johnson S. Lasko L.A. Baratz M. Gahlot V. Ehrlich G.D. Kathju S. Direct demonstration of viable Staphylococcus aureus biofilms in an infected total joint arthroplasty. A case report. J. Bone Joint Surg. Am. 2008;90:1751–1758. [PubMed: 18676908]

[61] Khalil H. Williams R.J. Stenbeck G. Henderson B. Meghji S. Nair S.P. Invasion of bone cells by Staphylococcus epidermidis. Microbes Infect. 2007;9:460–465. [PubMed: 17331787]

[62] Mitchell G. Lamontagne C.A. Brouillette E. Grondin G. Talbot B.G. Grandbois M. Malouin F. Staphylococcus aureus SigB activity promotes a strong fibronectin-bacterium interaction which may sustain host tissue colonization by small-colony variants isolated from cystic fibrosis patients. Mol. Microbiol. 2008;70:1540–1555. [PubMed: 19007412]

[63] Mahalingam D. Szegezdi E. Keane M. Jong S. Samali A. TRAIL receptor signalling and modulation: Are we on the right TRAIL? Cancer Treat. Rev. 2009;35:280–288. [PubMed: 19117685]

[64] Reott M.A. Ritchie-Miller S.L. Anguita J. Hudson M.C. TRAIL expression is induced in both osteoblasts containing intracellular Staphylococcus aureus and uninfected osteoblasts in infected cultures. FEMS Microbiol. Lett. 2008;278:185–192. [PubMed: 18070069]

[65] von Eiff C. Peters G. Becker K. The small colony variant (SCV) concept – the role of staphylococcal SCVs in persistent infections. Injury 2006;37(Suppl. 2):S26–S33. [PubMed: 16651068]

[66] Sendi P. Proctor R.A. Staphylococcus aureus as an intracellular pathogen: the role of small colony variants. Trends Microbiol. 2009;17:54–58. [PubMed: 19162480]

[67] von Eiff C. Staphylococcus aureus small colony variants: a challenge to microbiologists and clinicians. Int. J. Antimicrob. Agents 2008;31:507–510. [PubMed: 18180148]

[68] Fink B, Makowiak C, Fuerst M, Berger I, Schäfer P, Frommelt L. The value of synovial biopsy, joint aspiration and C-reactive protein in the diagnosis of late periprosthetic infection of total knee replacements. J Bone Joint Surg Br 2008;90:874–8. [PubMed: 18591595]

[69] Greidanus NV, Masri BA, Garbuz DS, et al. Use of erythrocyte sedimentation rate and C-reactive protein level to diagnose infection before revision total knee arthroplasty: a prospective evaluation.J Bone Joint Surg Am 2007;89:1409–16. [PubMed: 17606776]

[70] Müller M, Morawietz L, Hasart O, Strube P, Perka C, Tohtz S. Diagnosis of periprosthetic infection following total hip arthroplasty — evaluation of the diagnostic values of pre- and intraoperative parameters and the associated strategy to preoperatively select patients with a high probability of joint infection. J Orthop Surg 2008;3:31.

[71] Love C, Marwin SE, Palestro CJ. Nuclear medicine and the infected joint replacement. Semin Nucl Med 2009;39:66–78. [PubMed: 19038601]

[72] Kwee TC, Kwee RM, Alavi A. FDG-PET for diagnosing prosthetic joint infection: systematic review and metaanalysis. Eur J Nucl Med Mol Imaging 2008;35:2122–32. [PubMed: 18704405]

[73] Schinsky MF, Della Valle CJ, Sporer SM, Paprosky WG. Perioperative testing for joint infection in patients undergoing revision total hip arthroplasty. J Bone Joint Surg Am 2008;90:1869–75. [PubMed: 18762646]

[74] Cabrita H, Croci A, De Camargo O, De Lima A. Prospective study of the treatment of infected hip arthroplasties with or without the use of an antibiotic-loaded spacer. Clinics (Sao Paulo) 2007;62:99– 108. [PubMed: 17505692]

[75] Whittaker JP, Warren RE, Jones RS, Gregson PA. Is prolonged systemic antibiotic treatment essential in two-stage revision hip replacement for chronic Gram-positive infection? J Bone Joint Surg Br 2009;91:44–51. [Erratum, J Bone Joint Surg Br 2009;91:700.]. [PubMed: 19092003]

[76] Stockley I, Mockford BJ, Hoad-Red-dick A, Norman P. The use of two-stage exchange arthroplasty with depot antibiotics in the absence of long-term antibiotic therapy in infected total hip replacement. J Bone Joint Surg Br 2008;90:145–8. [PubMed: 18256078]

[77] Bratzler DW, Houck PM. Antimicrobial prophylaxis for surgery: an advisory statement from the National Surgical Infection Prevention Project. Am J Surg 2005;189:395– 404. [PubMed: 15820449]

[78] Xin-Yi Yang. Cong-Ran Li. Ren-Hui Lou. et al. In vitro activity of recombinant lysostaphin against Staphylococcus aureus isolates from hospitals in Beijing, China. Journal of Medical Microbiology (2007), 56, 71–76.

4

Arthroplasty in HIV/SCD Carriers

J. Bahebeck, D. Handy Eone, B. Ngo Nonga and T. Kingue Njie

University Hospitals of Yaoundé
Cameroun

1. Introduction

Due to the growing of HIV pandemic in the world and especially in Africa during the last two decades, it has become more and more frequent to find HIV infected patients with an absolute indication of arthroplasty. In fact, the indication of arthroplasty in these patients may be a very challenging issue. Even though all of these patients are not immune depressed, due to the known natural history of HIV carriage, the risk of future immune depression remain and logically the risk of immediate, early, or late infection of arthroplastic implants and subsequent loosening or worse, generalized infection. The literature on this question remains very scarce ; the first section of this chapter will present a classification of HIV carriers elected to Arthroplasty, describe protective measures for each class of patients, and present immediate , short and mid term expected results, based an a systematic analysis, and Authors own experience. The second section will be focused on arthroplasty in sickle cell disease (SCD) carriers, as these types of patients usually demand arthroplasty at the end stage of secondary vascular necrosis, the most frequent adult joint complication of their genetic condition. Lastly, as Very few, if any, is known in case where both conditions (HIV & SCD) are combined in the same patient demanding arthroplasty, a short section will be proposed.

Section A: Arthroplasty in HIV carriers

- Introduction
- Pathogenesis of HIV infection
- Work up and classification of HIV carriers elected for arthroplasty
- General principles & practices of antiretroviral therapy
- Antiretroviral therapy in HIV carriers demanding arthroplasty
- Prophylactic antibiotic therapy in HIV carriers undergoing arthroplasty
- Section A Summary

Due to the spreading of HIV worldwide during the latest decades, it had become more and more frequent in the orthopaedic practice, to indicate an arthroplasty, especially of the hip, in patients living with HIV. This virus has been incriminated by many authors as a possible causal agent in the case of bone's aseptic necrosis. The profiles of the HIV infected patients are variable: some are previous known carriers, other are discovered at the time of the preoperative workup. The duration of the preoperative antiretroviral treatment vary also from one patient to another. Anyhow, the main question for the orthopedic surgeon is to find out what is the level of the immune system of a person living with HIV and who is a candidate for an arthroplasty? In another words, what is the infection risk of the implant, whether immediately, in the short, the mid and even the long term? These questions may be better understood through a review of the pathogenesis of HIV infection.

1.1 Pathogenesis of HIV Infection

HIV infection is due to the introduction of the related virus in the body mainly through unprotected sexual intercourses, secondly through blood transfusion, and more rarely through other ways. Sometimes the patient may present a minor inflammatory syndrome lasting for few days with a complete recovery and no detectable virus for a long period. In some people, the virus will spread into the body fluids and organs and will slowly, but surely, destroy a specific type of lymphocytes, named CD4; the problem is that, CD4 are the hard ware of the body immune system and thus, the protector against numerous common infectious agents. With time, and after many years, no matter the apparent normal clinical state, the CD4 lymphocytes count which is normally above 500 Cells/Ml, will decrease progressively with a proportional depression of the HIV carrier immunity. If nothing is done, the general status of the patient will decompensate with severe weight loss, anemia and fatigue. He will develop opportunistic infections or tumors which are exceptional in an immune competent person. The most common opportunistic diseases are from the skull to the foot: brain toxoplasmosis, mouth and esophageal candidiasis, lung tuberculosis and pneumocystoses, intestinal cryptosporidiosis, leg and generalized Kaposi angiosarcomas, and various lymphomas. At this stage, the majority of patients are killed by a combination of these diseases and their complications. It is obvious that clinical pictures of HIV carriers are numerous, depending on the level of the immune depression; a classification is therefore necessary. The WHO-AIDS has proposed such a classification based both on the clinical picture and biological markers. However, as far as arthroplasty is concerned, the extreme majority of demanders of this surgery look clinically well; therefore, except in case where they declare themselves, if a systematic sample of HIV serologogy is not done, the surgeon may be taking the risk of a major surgical procedure in an advanced immune depressed patient. In our practice where the HIV carriage is up to 10% into the general population, HIV screening is mandatory before any elective arthroplasty. No matter the result, the benefice is defendable. In fact, in one hand, negative patients may at least undergo an auto transfusion program while, in the other hand, virus carriers will be classified and appropriately managed before or during arthroplasty. Such classification is mainly based on immunological work up, since, as it had been said above, quite all patients look healthy.

1.2 Work up and classification of HIV carriers elected for arthroplasty

After the diagnosis is done and an indication of arthroplasty is made, especially into the areas of high HIV carriage in the general population, the Orthopedic Surgeon should obtain an inform consent from his patient about this uncomfortable matter. In twelve years practice in our community, we have not had any of our patients for hip arthrosplasty resisting to the above arguments, but as with all medical information, discretion is the rule. If the patient is a known HIV carrier already on antiretroviral treatment, we will look up for his latest CD4 count and viral load. In the other cases, the screening is mandatory; if the patient is seronegative, he is managed conventionally with the advantage of auto transfusion program, provided hepatitis B and C serology are negative. In HIV positive screened patients, the next step is the confirmation western-Blot test; if the latest is negative; the patient is qualified as non HIV carrier and managed as usual. In case of confirmed HIV carriage by western-Blot test, the next step is the CD4 lymphocytes count and the viral load measurement by up to date procedures. The CD4 lymphocyte count is the key point for HIV carriers classification. Patients with less than 500 CD4 lymphocytes / ML are considered immune depressed and named **class A arthroplasty demanders.** Depending on whether this count is above 300, les than 300 with no opportunistic disease, or less than 300 with an opportunistic disease, Class A patients are further sub divided **A1, A2 or A3.** Non immune depressed HIV seropositive Patients with low infection risk are classified B; if they were known before and under treatment, they are sub-divided **B1,** if they have more than 500 CD4/ML with no treatment, they are sub-divided **B2.** This makes a total of 5 classes of arthroplasty demanders living with the virus (**B1, B2, A1, A2, A3**) and thus, who need specific protective measures and especially, antiretroviral therapy (ARVT).

1.3 General principles of antiretroviral therapy

Antiretroviral therapy (ARVT) was introduced in the early nineties with the aim to act against the multiplication of the HIV and therefore, to stop the destruction of the CD4 lymphocytes and subsequent immune depression. The drugs are numerous, but have been considered based on their action into 3 main classes which are: antiproteasis, nucleoside inhibitor of reverse transcriptases and non nucleoside inhibitor of reverse transcriptase. Into the middle of the decade, it clearly appeared that none of these classes could solely stop the viral replication and that, in the contrary, the triple combination was efficient. Shortly after, the common presentation became a triple antiretroviral fixed combination drugs commonly named TRITHERAPY.

There are two most common combinations that are: Efavirenz, Zidovudine and Lamivudine into one hand, and on the other hand, Niverapine, Stadivudine and Lamivudine. In case of drug resistance, a second line combination of Indinavir, Zidovudine and Lamivudine is proposed. The first line treatment, which is commonly used, has shown that besides few sides effects seen at the beginning of the treatment, that combination is usually well tolerated thereafter and it is efficient. In a large majority of patients the CD4 level will rise above 500/ML after weeks to months and the virus will be undetectable in the peripheral blood, making them significantly less contagious to their sexual partners. Many institutions in our country give drugs only to severely immune depressed carriers defined as AIDS patients. Moderately immune depressed and non immune depressed carriers are not treated. Therefore, it remained a question weather this policy does not favor the spreading of the disease through the world? Anyway, whenever an arhtroplasty is demanded by a HIV carrier, a different protocol of ARVT should be associated.

1.4 Antiretroviral therapy in HIV carriers demanding arthroplasty

Finally, 5 types of HIV carriers have been considered among arthroplasty demanders; they may need a similar number of protocols regarding ARVT.

1. **B1** Arthroplasty demanders are already known as HIV carriers and under ARVT; they should never stop their treatment even the day before and after surgery. There is nothing to do more, compare to non carriers patients. Exceptionally, if their CD4 count is low, they are referred to their physician to find out if this low count is due to drug resistance or to a non compliant attitude. The surgery should be delayed, and the issue corrected by a second line protocol ARVT.

2. Type **B2** arthroplasty demanders (HIV carriers with >500 CD4 lymphocytes/ML): they are not immune depressed no matter their viral load; they should be managed

according to the protocol of their physicians. Into our own practice, they will be operated with no ARVT and will be placed on treatment only if the CD4 count fall below 500/ML during the follow-up. After they have started with ARVT, they will continue it forever.

3. Type **A1** patients, (HIV carriers with 300 to 499 CD4 lymphocytes/ML), as they are moderately immune depressed, should be placed on ARVT shortly after the CD4 count results and they should undergo surgery without delay. Although it is not recommend by the official policy, we believe that they do need treatment before they undergo major surgery to give them a protection which may be needed anyway in the future.

4. Type **A2** arthroplasty demanders (HIV carriers with less than 300 CD4 lymphocytes/ML , but with no opportunistic disease), who are by definition asymptomatic, but severely immune depressed, are placed on ARVT and their surgery postponed for a few weeks till the CD4 lymphocytes/ML above 300 is obtained. Exceptionally in the emergency setting, the arthroplasty should not be postponed but the patient must be protected by a prolonged antibioprophylaxis which is actually an antibiotherapy.

5. Type **A3** arthroplasty demanders (HIV carriers with less than 300 CD4 lymphocytes/ML, but with an opportunistic disease) are first treated for their opportunistic disease, various prophylaxes, ARVT and the surgery postponed as above.

In all the cases, prophylactic antibiotic therapy should also be considered.

1.5 Prophylactic antibiotic therapy in HIV carriers undergoing arthroplasty

The aim of classical **prophylactic antibiotic therapy** (**PATB**) is to keep the surgical site under antibiotic protection during the short period of decrease immune response around the perioperative period. This period, which is less than 72 hours in a normal individual, may be prolonged in cases of immune depressed HIV carriers. Our previous study has shown that there is no significant difference in rates of post-operative infections between immune depressed and non immune depressed patients when we extend **PATB** to 10 ten days ,what we call **prolonged prophylactic antibiotherapy**, (**PPATB**) as one would expect. Although there were only few cases of arthroplasty in this serie. Finally, as far as arthroplasty demanders are concerned, two different regiments of prophylactic antibiotic therapy are to be considered, that is:

1. The classical regiment of PATB with intravenous cefuroxime (or any other second generation cephalosporin); 1.5g at the anesthesia induction, followed by 750 mg every 12h within not more than 72 hours. This is indicated for class B arthroplasty demanders.

2. The extended regiment of **PPATB** into which the   above regiment is maintained during 10 days. This is indicated for all class A arthroplasty demanders.

1.6 Section A summary

Finally, combined protective measures of HIV carriers demanding atrhroplasty may be summarized as follow (table I), depending of their classification:

1. B2 patients should continue their previous ARVT and, get normal PABT during the arthroplasty which should not be delayed.

2. B1 may wait to start ARVT when the CD4 count will cross the 500 line; they should undergo normal PABT and their arthroplasty with no delay.

3. A1 patients should start an ARVT and get their arthroplasty not delayed but under protective PPABT.

4. A2 patients should start the ARVT and the arthroplasty delayed when they cross the 300 line in their CD4 count; the surgery should be protected by a PPABT.
5. A3 patient should first be treated for their opportunist disease and later on managed as A2.

With these measures, we think that the results of arthroplasty in HIV carriers should be comparable to HIV seronegative counterparts.

	Definition	ARVT?	PABT?	PPABT?
B1	HIV +, under ARVT	YES	YES	NO
B2	HIV+, CD4>500	NO	YES	NO
A1	HIV+, 300<CD4<500	YES	NO	YES
A2	HIV+, CD4<300 no opportunist infection-	YES	NO	YES
A3	HIV+,CD4<300 & some opportunist infection	YES	NO	YES

Table 1. Summarizing the use of ARVT, PABT, & PPABT in the five type HIV carriers demanders of arthroplasty

2. Section B: Arthroplasty in SCD carriers

- Definition & history of SCD
- Physiopathology of SCD & related secondary avascular necrosis
- Diagnosis and classification of SCD
- Work-up and management of SCD systemic acute complications
- Section B summary

2.1 Definition & history of SCD

SCD is a chronic hemolytic hemoglobinopathy that is genetically transmitted. During a crisis, red blood cells become sickle-shaped increasing blood viscosity, slowing blood flow, and consequently plugging small blood vessels creating widespread thromboembolic tissue infarction.

This genetic disease which is the most frequent genetic disease in black people, is also the most common cause of femoral head necrosis in them. In fact, SCD touches up to 0·74% of the births in sub-Saharan Africa, while this number is 10-20 times less in Europe and North America. In Nigeria, an estimated 45,000 to 90,000 babies are born each year with SCD. The African blacks are the main victims but the disease is also distributed in the south of Italy, Greece, Turkey, the Arabian Gulf, especially Saudi Arabia, and the Indian subcontinent. In the United States SCD occurs in approximately 1 out of every 500 African American births. People in the USA with sickle-cell disease number 90,000 of which 80,000 are black and 10,000 are Hispanic. The state with the highest sickle-cell population was New York with 8000, followed by Florida with 7500, and Texas with 6700 people with SCD. FLOUZAT-LACHANIETTE et al. report a series of SCD patients developing secondary avascular necrosis that originated from Africa, the United States of America, the Indian subcontinent, the Persian Gulf and from Mediterranean countries. Multifocal secondary vascular necrosis was found to occur in at least 64 percent of patients.

2.2 Physiopathology of SCD & related secondary avascular necrosis

Herrick first described the characteristic sickle-shaped erythrocytes in 1910 and Pauling and colleagues identified the abnormal hemoglobin (HbS) and coined the term "molecular disease" in 1949 . Hemoglobin A is normally found in the adult and is composed of four globular protein subunits the α and β globins. A fetal form or hemoglobin F is also found, normally, in small proportion in the adult. In SCD, an inappropriate substitution of valine for glutamine at the sixth position of the β globin chain produces hemoglobin S that polymerizes at low oxygen tensions. This causes the red cell to sickle which increases viscosity in the microvasculature and leads recurrent episodes of vaso-occlusion. These recurring episodes of widespread infarcts in patients homozygous for the sickle cell gene (HbSS) cause life-threatening conditions such as renal failure, acute chest syndrome, autosplenectomy, immune deficiency and infection all leading to an early death. As far as heavy surgery and especially arthroplasty is concerned in SCD patients; the key points and the difference with non SCD patients will therefore be focused into the prevention, the monitoring, and if needed, the management of the above cited acute systemic complications.

But SCD complications are not just acute; these repeated cycles of hypoxia and inflammation due to sickling cause chronic musculo-skeletal pain and finally secondary avascular necrosis of bone ends, especially, femoral and humeral heads, and less frequently, femoral condyles. This secondary avascular necrosis, at the end stages, causes severe chronic joints pain and functional impairment, for which very few solutions except of arthroplasties are currently available. In deed, secondary avascular necrosis is the leading indication of arthroplasty in SCD carriers. Secondary avascular necrosis doesn't occur only in homozygous HbSS patients; it is also common in heterozygous SCD clinically asymptomatic carriers with AS hemoglobin. In to the other hand, other types of abnormal hemoglobin such as HbC (Substitution of a lysine for glutamine at the 6th position of the β-globin chain) are also found in some patients with similar effects. Finally, secondary avasular necrosis due to SCD is therefore not exclusively observed in homozygous SS patients (HbSS); it should also be suspected in various other heterozygous forms; especially, HbAS and HbSC carriers.

2.3 Diagnosis and classification of SCD and related secondary avascular necrosis

To specifically diagnose SCD, cheap and widely available techniques such as hemoglobin electrophoresis or chromatography accurately determine the levels of HbA, HbF, HbS and HbC.

For secondary avascular necrosis and bony lesions due to SCD, standard X-ray, C-T Scan, Isotope Scan, and MRI are indicated in various stages for diagnosis and staging. However, the FICAT- ARLET classification is the must commonly used world wide. It is divided in four stages as below.

FICAT-ARLET classification of AVN (17):

Stage I: MRI changes

Stage II: Sclerotic and cystic changes
Stage III :   Collapse
Stage IV: Osteoarthritis on both sides

2.4 Work-up and management of SCD systemic acute complications
2.4.1 General
Preoperatively the HbS level should be of less than 30% of the circulating hemoglobin before major surgery such as Arthroplasty; however, VICHINSKY et al., have shown in a randomized controlled trial that, exchange transfusion may not be necessary to avoid complications. In all cases, it is prudent to take the preoperative hemoglobin concentration to 100 g/L and to keep it at this level in the early postoperative phase; this objective may be obtained by ordinary transfusion of normal red blood cells as it may be confirmed by post transfusion electrophoresis or chromatography. This will also reduce the risk of peri-operative thromboembolic complications. The above target hemoglobin level may be rich by preoperative oral folic acid of few weeks, in those SCD patients with less than 30% of HbSS during the initial work-up; however, at least postoperatively, blood transfusion will be needed. It should be clear that, to the best of current literature, there is no place for autologous blood transfusion in SCD patients; these patients should always be managed with homologous bank blood products. In the other hand, Reduction of HbS concentrations may be obtained by the chronically use of hydroxycarbamide because this increases the concentration of fetal hemoglobin (HbF) which reduces hemolysis and prevents vaso-occlusion. It is also well known that that hypothermia, acidosis, hypoxemia and dehydration should be avoided pre and postoperatively.

2.4.2 Acute chest syndrome
Acute chest syndrome is a specificity of SCD and affects around 20% of the patients. A combination of thoracic pain, fever and infiltrates on thoracic x-ray characterizes this syndrome. The etiology is multifactorial including pulmonary embolism, microvascular occlusion and infection Severity varies, but 13% of patients require mechanical ventilation and 3% may die. In a post operative period of any arthroplasty procedure in SCD patient, this syndrome should be seriously considered in establishing etiologies of acute chest pain. In fact, it prevention and management include respiratory support, antibiotics, blood transfusions and deep venous thromboses prophylaxis/therapy. At times corticosteroids may be indicated.

2.4.3 Infection
Susceptibility to infection is an issue in SCD. Many of these patients are immunocompromised because of autosplenectomy and osteonecrotic tissues tend to be colonized by Gram negative organisms. Several organisms have been identified as important causes of infection including S pneumoniae, H influenza, and non-typhi Salmonella species and appropriate antibiotic prophylaxis and immunization must be instituted in these patients. Therefore, a systematic preoperative investigation should be undertaken prior to any Arthroplasty procedure in a SCD patient to rule out occult infection; this should a least include urine culture, ENT consultation and dental examination and corrections. If there is a suspicion of infectious foyers a full antibiotic

treatment should be undertaken with normalization of biological markers prior to the joint procedure. After arthroplasty, bone fragments from joint resection and reaming should also be send for bacterial analysis; if positive, a specific antibiotic testing should be undertaken. Subsequently, a long term antibiotic therapy should be undertaken in collaboration with the infectious diseases team, and till the normalization of biological infectious markers.

2.5 Section B summary

Finally, arthroplasties of the Hip, the knee, the shoulder or any other joint may commonly be demanded by SCD patients, mainly due the high frequency secondary avascular necrosis as a chronic complication of their genetic condition. The procedure may be performed with at least acceptable results, provided the following precautions are properly taken:

- Conventional biological work-up and especially, the hemoglobin types/ratios, and comprehensive research of occult infections.
- Preoperative treatment of any occult or evident infection
- Enhancement of the fetal hemoglobin ratio by chronic preoperative administration of hydroxycarbamide.
- Enhancement of the total Hemoglobin level to 100G/ml preoperatively, by chronic oral folic acid, and maintaining it so per and post operatively by homologous red blood cells
- Optimal oxygenation during the early post operative period
- Optimal fluid infusion during the early post-operative period
- Adequate warming during the early post-operative period
- Avoiding any acidosis state by blood gas control and correction during the early post operative period
- Culture of bone resection/reaming products and subsequent long standing and targeted post arthroplasty antibiotic therapy
- Avoiding autologous blood transfusion

3. Section C: Arthroplasty in HIV & SCD carriers

- Introduction
- HIV carriage in SCD patients
- Antiretroviral therapy in SCD patients
- Summary of section C

3.1 Introduction

After sexual intercourse, blood transfusion had been considered as one the possible pathway HIV contamination. Into the other hand, due acute episodes and chronic anemia, SCD patient had been to be more frequently transfused than normal hemoglobin carriers; it therefore appear rational to hypothesize that SCD patients present a higher risk of HIV infection. The literature on this matter is very scars; and the clinical experience does not confirm this theorical thinking.This may be due to at least a reduction on the transfusion rate in sickles and a better safety of blood banking systems. In the other hand, both HIV &

SCD have been incriminated as high risk factor or secondary aseptic necrosis, mainly of the hip. Provided the standard treatment of aseptic necrosis of the Hip is total hip arthroplasty, it become evident although rare and not reported currently, combination of both condition (SCD& HIV) in patients demanding arthroplasty, may in the next future, become a challenging issue. There is no evidence base on this precise issue; however, since the above both section A and B have been focused respectively on arthroplasty in HIV carriers in one hand, and in another one, Arthroplasty in SCD, knowing about HIV carriage in SCD patients may help to set up our thinking regarding arthroplasty in patients with both conditions.

3.2 HIV carriage in SCD patients

As it has been said above, the literature on HIV carriage in SCD patients is very scars, due to the paucity of patients themselves. In fact, the clinical experience in Central Africa where HIV carriage is higher than 10% in general population, shows that this rate is not significantly higher in homozygous HbSS patients. Further more, as the large majority of HbSS homozygous patients are also sexually active, it make sense to believe that the HIV infection in these specific set, is got through the same pathways with the general population. One of the rare related paper we could found regarding this matter is the one of Bagasra O et al; it suggests that, in patients with both SS and HIV-1 infection, the retroviral disease may be ameliorated by host factors of which absence of splenic function prior to HIV-1 contamination may be one. In another term, this author assume that HbSS carriage makes the body more resistant to HIV process as into his experimental case-control study of ten years follow-up, both the CD4 count and the Viral load were better in HbSS patients with HIV infection compare to HbAA counter part with the same viral infection. This may be explained by the fact that, as the spleen and lymph nodes are major sites of human immunodeficiency virus type 1 replication, mutation, and genetic variation in vivo; and as a major portion of this lymphatic tissue, such as the spleen, is removed or otherwise is unavailable for invasion by the HIV-1 virus, the course of this infection is altered. The clinical consequence is a prolonged symptom-free interval or even increased survival that we experience in daily clinical follow up of homozygous HbSS patients. Into the contrary, as it was reported by Sellier P et al, no significant difference in HIV infection progression is observed between heterozygous SCD carriers with HIV and their normal Hemoglobin counter part with the same virus.

Therefore, as far as HIV carriage is concerned in SCD patients, we should always distinguish homozygous patients in which, the expected course of retroviral process is slow than usual in one side, and in the other side, heterozygous patient in which it does not differ from that of the non SCD-non HIV patients. The same differentiation may be necessary regarding the management of antiretroviral therapy (ARVT) in this field.

3.3 Antiretroviral therapy in SCD patients

If we agree to distinguish Homozygous patients from their heterozygous counterpart regarding the HIV carriage, it makes sense to do the same in the matter of ARVT.

Regarding first homozygous HbSS patients, to the best of our knowledge, no evidence exist on the use of ARVT on them. However, on observing a short cohort of 5 patients in our practice at the Central Hospital of Yaoundé in Cameroun in to the last 5 years, our standard protocol of ARVT has been well tolerated by homozygous HbSS patients, provided all the other measures of SCD control are well conducted.

In the contrary, we have more heterozygous SCD patients with HIV carriage under ARVT; as said above; the tolerance and efficiency of ARVT on them does not differ from the general non SCD population.

3.4 Summary of section C

There is very little evidences and experience on how to manage patients demanding arthroplasty, in cases where they are simultaneously HIV and SCD carriers. This little experience shows that those who are heterozygous should be managed as non SCD patients. In those who are homozygous, a simultaneous protocol of SCD care protocol as presented in section B, should be added.

4. References

[1] Bagasra O, Steiner RM, Ballas SK, Castro O, Dornadula G, Embury S, Jungkind D, Bobroski L, Kutlar A, Burchott S. Viral burden and disease progression in HIV-1-infected patients with sickle cell anemia. Am J Hematol. 1998 Nov;59(3):199-207

[2] J. Bahebeck a,*, D. Handy Eone b, B. Ngo Nonga c, T. Ndjie Kingue d, M. Sosso: Implant orthopaedic surgery in HIV asymptomatic carriers: Management and early outcome. Injury, Int. J. Care Injured 40 (2009) 1147–1150.

[3] Bahebeck J,. Atangana R, Techa A, Monny-Lobe M, Sosso M, Hoffmeyer P. Relative rates and features of musculoskeletal complications in adult sicklers. Acta Orthop Belg 2004, 70(2): 107-111.

[4] Brousseau DC, Panepinto JA, Nimmer M, Hoffmann RG. The number of people with sickle-cell disease in the United States: national and state estimates. Am J Hematol. 2010 Jan;85(1):77-8.

[5] Ficat RP, Arlet J. Functional investigation of bone under normal conditions. In: Ficat RP, Arlet J, Hungerford DS (eds): Ischemia and necroses of bone. Baltimore, MD, Williams and Wilkins. 1980. 29-52.

[6] Flouzat-Lachaniette CH, Roussignol X, Poignard A, Mukasa MM, Manicom O, Hernigou P. Multifocal joint osteonecrosis in sickle cell disease. Open Orthop J. 2009,15;3:32-5.

[7] Gutierrez F, Padilla S, Masia M, et al. Osteonecrosis in patients infected with HIV: clinical epidemiology and natural history in a large case series from Spain. J Acquir Immune Defic Syndr. 2006;42(3):286–292. [PubMed]

[8] Harrison WJ, Lewis CP, Lavy CB. Wound healing after implant surgery in HIV-positive patients. J Bone Joint Surg Br. 2002;84(6):802–806. [PubMed]

[9] Hernigou P, Zilber S, Filippini P, Mathieu G, Poignard A, Galacteros F. Total THA in adult osteonecrosis related to sickle cell disease. Clin Orthop Relat Res 2008, 466(2): 300-308.

[10] Hoekman P, van de Perre P, Nelissen J, Kwisanga B, Bogaerts J, Kanyangabo F. Increased frequency of infection after open reduction of fractures in patients who

are seropositive for human immunodeficiency virus. J Bone Joint Surg Am. 1991;73(5):675–679. [PubMed]

[11] Jeong Joon Yoo, Sae Hyung Chun,Young Sam Kwon, Kyung-Hoi Koo, Kang Sup Yoon, Hee Joong Kim. Operations about Hip in Human Immunodeficiency Virus-Positive Patients. Clin Orthop Surg. 2010 March; 2(1): 22–27.

[12] Keruly JC, Chaisson RE, Moore RD. Increasing inicidence of avascular necrosis of the hip in HIV-infected patients. J Acquir Immune Defic Syndr. 2001;28(1):101–102. [PubMed]

[13] Lehman CR, Ries MD, Paiement GD, Davidson AB. Infection after total joint arthroplasty in patients with human immunodeficiency virus or intravenous drug use. J Arthroplasty. 2001;16(3):330–335. [PubMed]

[14] Mahoney CR, Glesby MJ, DiCarlo EF, Peterson MG, Bostrom MP. Total hip arthroplasty in patients with human immunodeficiency virus infection: pathologic findings and surgical outcomes. Acta Orthop. 2005;76(2):198–203. [PubMed]

[15] Miller KD, Masur H, Jones EC, et al. High prevalence of osteonecrosis of the femoral head in HIV-infected adults. Ann Intern Med. 2002;137(1):17–25. [PubMed]

[16] Morse CG, Mican JM, Jones EC, et al. The incidence and natural history of osteonecrosis in HIV-infected adults. Clin Infect Dis. 2007;44(5):739–748. [PubMed]

[17] Paiement GD, Hymes RA, LaDouceur MS, Gosselin RA, Green HD. Postoperative infections in asymptomatic HIV-seropositive orthopedic trauma patients. J Trauma. 1994;37(4):545–550. [PubMed]

[18] Parvizi J, Sullivan TA, Pagnano MW, Trousdale RT, Bolander ME. Total joint arthroplasty in human immunodeficiency virus-positive patients: an alarming rate of early failure. J Arthroplasty. 2003;18(3):259–264. [PubMed]

[19] Platt OS, Brambilla DJ, Rosse WF et al. Mortality in sickle cell disease : life expectancy and risk factors for early death. N Engl J Med. 1994;330:1639-44

[20] Rees DC, Williams TN ,Gladwin MT. Sickle-cell disease. Lancet 2010; 376: 2018–31.

[21] Ries MD, Barcohana B, Davidson A, Jergesen HE, Paiement GD. Association between human immunodeficiency virus and osteonecrosis of the femoral head. J Arthroplasty. 2002;17(2):135–139. [PubMed]

[22] Scribner AN, Troia-Cancio PV, Cox BA, et al. Osteonecrosis in HIV: a case-control study. J Acquir Immune Defic Syndr. 2000;25(1):19–25. [PubMed]

[23] Sellier P, Masson E, Zini JM, Simoneau G, Magnier JD, Evans J, Bergmann JF : Disease progression in HIV-1-infected patients heterozygous for the sickle hemoglobin gene. AIDS. 2009 Nov 13;23(17):2362-4.

[24] Taylor LE, Stotts NA, Humphreys J, Treadwell MJ, Miaskowski C. A review of the literature on the multiple dimensions of chronic pain in adults with sickle cell disease. J Pain Symptom Manage. 2010;40(3):416-35.

[25] Vichinsky EP, Haberkern CM, Neumayr L, Earles AN, Black D, Koshy M, Pegelow C, Abboud M, Ohene-Frempong K, Iyer RV. A comparison of conservative and aggressive transfusion regimens in the perioperative management of sickle cell disease. The Preoperative Transfusion in Sickle Cell Disease Study Group. N Engl J Med. 1995;333:206–213.

[26] Vichinsky EP, Neumayr LD, Earles AN, Williams R, Lennette ET, Dean D, Nickerson B, Orringer E, McKie V, Bellevue R, Daeschner C, Manci EA. Causes and outcomes of the acute chest syndrome in sickle cell disease. National Acute Chest Syndrome Study Group. N Engl J Med, 2000;342:1855–1865.

Part 2

Arthroplasty of Spine and Upper Extremity

5

Lumbar Spinal Arthroplasty: Clinical Experience

Fred H. Geisler

Chicago Back Institute, Swedish Covenant Hospital, N. Francisco, Chicago, IL
USA

1. Introduction

Lumbar spinal arthroplasty was first reported in clinical settings more than 10 years ago by Griffith et al [1]. This early experience was acquired with the first lumbar artificial disc, the CHARITÉ I, in patients with degenerative disc disease. Since that time, a randomized controlled trial comparing arthroplasty with the CHARITÉ Artificial Disc vs. anterior lumbar interbody fusion with the BAK Cage and iliac crest bone was completed. Multiple other lumbar arthroplasty devices have been developed subsequent to the CHARITÉ and are undergoing or completing clinical trials.

Unlike other spinal medical devices, lumbar discs are required by the Food and Drug Administration to complete randomized controlled trials (RCT) prior to market approval in the United States. As a result, lumbar arthroplasty devices have undergone more scrutiny and clinical evaluation than any other spinal medical devices. Specifically, a new device, the ProDisc-L, was granted FDA approval in 2006 and was described in a recent peer-review publication[2]. In addition, the Maverick Total Disc Arthroplasty System (Medtronic Sofamor Danek), Kineflex Lumbar Disc (SpinalMotion), and FlexiCore Intervertebral Disc (SpineCore/Stryker) lumbar discs have both completed their randomized enrollments and are currently in continued access (non-randomized) mode.

All these ongoing and completed randomized clinical trials have generated a large body of evidence on the safety and efficacy of arthroplasty for lumbar spine in clinical applications and, in many cases, in Level-1 publications.

The safety and efficacy of arthroplasty are not the only parameters discussed in the >60 clinical papers published over the last 6 years. In fact, significant insights were developed in the impact of arthroplasty on sagittal alignment and motion, possible adverse events and reoperation, as well as optimal patient selection and indication. Surgical technique and health economics papers have also been generated in an effort to fully understand the clinical and societal impact of this new technology. This review paper is aimed at providing an overview of all the existing clinical data related to spinal arthroplasty.

2. Materials and methods

A search was conducted on the OVID and COCHRANE Library database to collect all clinical data relevant to spinal arthroplasty. Specifically, the following keywords were used:

(CHARITÉ Artificial Disc or ProDisc-L or Maverick Total Disc Arthroplasty System or KineFlex or FlexiCore Intervertebral Disc) and (disc) and (lumbar). The search was limited to English-language papers. Preclinical, biomechanical, and review papers were excluded from the final paper selection. In addition, papers describing obsolete devices (CHARITÉ I and CHARITÉ II) were also excluded from the study. A total of 60 papers were analyzed herein and subdivided by key topic, as following: 1) General clinical outcomes; 2) Radiographic Analysis: Range of motion, heterotopic ossification and sagittal balance analyses; 3) facet and adjacent-level degeneration; 4) Revisions and revision strategies; 5) Surgical technique; 6) Complications; 7) Special patient population analyses; and 8) Health economics evaluations.

3. Results

3.1 General clinical outcome results

General clinical outcome results were available for the CHARITÉ Artificial Disc, the ProDisc-L, the Maverick Total Disc Arthroplasty System, and the FlexiCore Intervertebral Disc. However, level-1 data was only available for the CHARITÉ Artificial disc and the ProDisc-L, as the final study FDA IDE results for the Maverick Total Disc Arthroplasty System and the FlexiCore Intervertebral Disc have yet to be published.

The CHARITÉ Artificial Disc manuscripts described clinical outcomes as early as 1 year [3] and up to 13 years post-operative[4]. The short/medium term papers included herein typically disclosed early analyses from single sites involved in the CHARITÉ Artificial Disc IDE study comparing arthroplasty with CHARITÉ Artificial Disc vs. anterior interbody fusion with BAK cage and autograft [3, 5, 6]. The complete RCT at 2-year follow-up included 205 arthroplasty and 99 fusion patients, and was thoroughly described in two manuscripts, one focused on clinical outcomes[7], the other on radiographic outcomes[8]. Three additional medium- and long-term studies were also found: 2 papers with 10-year follow-up [4, 9] and one with an average of 6.6 year follow-up [10].

Safety and efficacy of arthroplasty was demonstrated in all short- and medium-term studies. Specifically, at 2-years post-operative, Blumenthal and McAfee reported no device-related complications and a reoperation rate of 5.4% (vs. 9.1% in the control arm). Efficacy was also demonstrated using validated disability (ODI) and pain (VAS) clinical outcomes tools. At 2 years, the reduction in ODI reached 48.5% (vs. 42.4% in the control group) and the absolute reduction in VAS reached 40.6 points (vs. 34.1 points in the control group) [7, 8].

Two of the three long-term studies confirmed these findings. Lemaire et al reported 10-year follow-up results in 100 patients. [4] This study included 54 patients operated at one level, 45 patients operated at two levels and one patient operated at 3 levels. Overall, authors reported excellent or good clinical outcomes in 90% cases. In a second long-term study, David et al presented 10-year data on 106 patients[9]. Only one-level surgeries were performed in this study. Excellent or good clinical outcome was obtained in 82.1% patients. Both papers thus concluded that arthroplasty was a viable option for disc degeneration.

Recently, a third, medium-term paper was published by Ross et al, describing the long-term effect of arthroplasty in 160 patients (226 CHARITÉ Artificial Discs). This paper reported a cumulative survival rate at 156 months of 35% and a mean ODI score improvement of 14%. Implant removal was also described in 12 patients[10]. These relatively poor findings were further discussed in two Letters to the Editors, which pointed out mathematical inconsistencies and overall clinical flaws in the manuscript, and further highlighted the need of proper surgical technique and patient selection for optimal clinical outcome [11, 12].

The ProDisc-L manuscripts described clinical outcomes as early as 3 months[13] and up to 8.7 years post-operative [14]. As described above for CHARITÉ Artificial Disc, The short-term papers typically disclosed early findings from one or two of the sites that participated in the randomized controlled trial comparing ProDisc-L against a 360 degree fusion[13, 15-21]. The complete RCT at 2-year follow-up included 161 arthroplasty and 75 fusion patients [2]. The long-term data included 64 patients operated at one site, of which 55 were available between 7 and 11 years post-operative, for clinical and radiographic follow-up[14]. All these studies concluded similarly that disc arthroplasty, at all evaluated time points, was safe and resulted in complication and/or re-operation rates comparable to those generally accepted for spinal surgery (complication rate of 9% at 8.7 years[14]; there were no major complications, but a reoperation rate of 3.7% at 2 years was reported[2]). In addition to safety, efficacy of spinal arthroplasty was also shown herein as all cases presented significant improvements in pain and disability. The final RCT data reported improvements in the arthroplasty group in Visual Analogue Scores (VAS) for pain by an average 39-mm, and in disability, as determined by the Oswestry Disability Index (ODI), by 28 points. It is worth noting, however, that the ODI tool utilized in this RCT was not the validated and widely accepted ODI methodology Version 1.0 as defined by Fairbanks et al[22]. In a Letter to the Editor, Fairbanks denounced the use of the so-called Oswestry Disability Index in the ProDisc-L study and thus cast doubt on the validity of the disability improvement outcomes observed herein[23].

The 2 clinical data publications on the MAVERICK device were both based on the same data set of 64 patients, collected at one site[24, 25]. The clinical outcomes were described using the ODI Version 1.0 and VAS scores. The efficacy of arthroplasty was once again demonstrated using these tools, as ODI scores decreased by an average of 20.7 points and VAS scores by 4.4 points. As for the FlexiCore Intervertebral Disc, only one paper was recently published[26]. This manuscript describes the clinical outcomes of 44 patients, of which only 6 were available for 2-year follow-up. While the clinical relevance of this data may therefore be questionable, authors still concluded that the device may be safe and efficacious but that the data was not representative of the entire patient cohort.

3.2 Radiographic analyses: Range of motion, heterotopic ossification and sagittal balance analyses

Radiographic evaluations such as ROM, heterotopic ossification, and sagittal balance have been broadly analyzed for the CHARITÉ Artificial Disc, the ProDisc-L, as well as the Maverick Total Disc Arthroplasty System.

Unlike other clinical and radiographic outcomes, accurate measurement of ROM was shown to be challenging and, to some extent, subjective, as patient positioning, imaging staff training, and other factors unrelated to the actual motion potential of the spine were shown to impact final readings [27]. Using ProDisc-L cases, Lim et al evaluated different methodologies and associated error margins for the measurement of ROM from radiographic images. Specifically, Lim et al concluded that a ROM of at least 4.6 degs must be observed in order to be 95% certain that a given device had any sagittal motion at all. Similarly, changes needed to be at least 9.6 degs in ROM in order to confirm at 95% that change in motion really happened[28, 29]. These technical limitations might explain the inconsistent ROM data, particularly for ProDisc-L cases, found in the published literature. The flexion-extension ROM results from the 2-year RCT were determined at 7.7 degrees and 4.67 degrees and characterized as a normal ROM [2]. However, at 8.7 years post-operative, Huang et al reported a ROM less than that reported in asymptomatic normal individuals, with an average motion of 3.8 degs [30]. In a 2006 prospective study on 41 patients with 2 year follow-up, Leivseth et al also reported that the device fails to restore normal segmental motion, while another retrospective study on 26 patients concluded that sagittal balance and ROM significantly improved after lumbar arthroplasty[31].

Less controversy was observed when reviewing ROM data for the CHARITÉ Artificial Disc. A complete manuscript was dedicated to the radiographic data of the 2-year RCT of the CHARITÉ Artificial Disc [8]. In this study, arthroplasty patients had a 13.6% increase in motion from preoperative to the 2-year post-operative time point. The ROM also correlated to device placement, as poor device placement resulted in a statistically significant reduction in motion. At 10-year follow-up, David reported an average 10.1 degs ROM, a value very similar to the 10.3 degs reported by Lemaire et al in their 10-year follow-up study[4, 9].

Le Huec et al published the only data available on radiographic findings after arthroplasty with the Maverick Total Disc Arthroplasty System. In their study, Le Huec et al broadened their analysis to include sagittal alignment and pelvic tilt[24, 32]. Using data related to 35 patients at an average 14 months post-operative, authors showed maintenance of overall lordosis and unchanged sacral and pelvic tilts, following arthroplasty.

More recently, a study by Tournier comparing all three - CHARITÉ Artificial Disc, ProDisc-L and Maverick Total Disc Arthroplasty System - further refined the analyses from LeHuec on pelvic and sagittal tilt. In this study, authors found no difference in ROM between prostheses and observed maintenance of sagittal balance before and after surgery with all devices. However, modifications of the lumbar curvature were observed[33].

The issue of heterotopic ossification in clinical cases of lumbar arthroplasty has been presented by McAfee et al and, more recently, by Tortolani et al[34, 35]. In his 2003 paper, McAfee introduced a novel method to characterize spinal heterotopic ossification. This methodology was applied by Tortolani et al in reviewing the 276 arthroplasty patients from the CHARITÉ Artificial Disc RCT (randomized and non-randomized cases). From this analysis, 4.3% cases of heterotopic ossification were noted. However, heterotopic ossification was not related to range of motion, as the authors concluded that no difference in the range of motionat 24-months post-operatively was found between the patients who had and those who did not have heterotopic ossification.

3.3 Facets and adjacent-level degeneration
Facet degeneration is currently a contraindication for arthroplasty. However, a few publications have investigated the impact of arthroplasty on index-level facet joints, as

well as adjacent-level discs, in order to determine whether the added motion at the index level could slow down the natural progression of the disease at the facets and the adjacent-level joints.

Three long-term analyses evaluated adjacent-level degeneration, one with ProDisc-L at 8.7 years, and the other two with the CHARITÉ Artificial Disc at 10 years follow-up. In the ProDisc-L study, 24% cases developed adjacent level degeneration by the latest follow-up time point. A correlation was also found between a low range of motion and the prevalence of adjacent level degeneration: all patients with adjacent-level degeneration had a ROM l ess than 5 degrees, while only 59% of patients without adjacent-level degeneration had a ROM less than 5 degrees [36]. Lemaire et al and David reported 2 (2%) and 3 (2.8%) cases of adjacent-level degeneration at the latest time point, respectively[4, 9]. Lemaire et al and David also disclosed 11 cases (11%) and 5 cases (4.7%) with facet arthrosis at the latest time point, respectively.

The issue of facet degeneration was also recently discussed in a short-term study. From a 13-patient case series with 12 months follow-up, Trouillier et al alluded to possible maintenance of facet joint integrity following arthroplasty with CHARITÉ Artificial Disc based on the favorable results from their series[37]. At the other end of the spectrum, Shim et al, at the 3-year time point, observed 36.4% and 32.0% increase in index-level facet degeneration and 19.4% and 28.6% adjacent level disc degeneration with the CHARITÉ Artificial Disc and the ProDisc-L, respectively.

3.4 Revision and revision strategies

The issue of possible revisability of arthroplasty devices represented a key concern when the first artificial disc, the CHARITÉ Artificial Disc, was introduced to the market. As such, multiple papers have focused on this issue and provided surgical and clinical insights to ensure appropriate approaches to revision surgery.

The first description of appropriate revision for a CHARITÉ Artificial Disc was presented by David[38]. In this single-case example, a CHARITÉ Artificial Disc was replaced at 9.5 years post-operative with another CHARITÉ Artificial Disc. The author concluded that revision of the disc with another disc could be safely and adequately performed and was thus an alternative to a revision fusion procedure. David also noted that, due to the inherent difficulty of an anterior approach, only experienced surgeons should undertake this operation. Further revision and explantation of the disc were also described by McAfee et al and Leary et al [39, 40]. McAfee et al confirmed Davids experience and concluded that arthroplasty with the CHARITÉ Artificial Disc did not preclude any further procedures at the index level during primary insertion, with nearly one third being revisable to a new motion-preserving prosthesis and just over two thirds being successfully converted to ALIF and/or posterior pedicle screw arthrodesis, the original alternative procedure. Leary further implied that technical errors in position and sizing of the implant were largely to blame for further revision surgery. Finally, Punt et al reviewed 75 revision cases from the Dutch experience (estimated by the authors at approximately more than 1000 Dutch patients). In this series, patients were fused posteriorly either with removal of the disc or without removal of the disc. No statistically significant difference was observed between these 2 groups[41]. This paper included patients previously described by Van Ooij et al[42].

3.5 Surgical technique

The appropriate surgical technique with the CHARITÉ Artificial Disc as well as the ProDisc-L was presented in 2 separate publications. Geisler et al provided a detailed account of the surgical technique for the CHARITÉ Artificial Disc, and dedicated an entire section of the paper to patient selection and preoperative planning, two critical aspects of successful spinal arthroplasty[43]. Authors also strongly recommended the availability of a spinal access surgeon to perform the approach, especially in revision cases. Finally, appropriate midline identification and positioning of the device also represented a critical discussion point in this paper. For the ProDisc-L, Gumbs et al retrospectively reviewed 64 cases of open retroperitoneal exposures and concluded that the approach was safe and, as discussed by Geisler et al, required a multidisciplinary team, such as an orthopedic and an access or general surgeon, to minimize complication rates[44].

3.6 Complications

Complications from spinal arthroplasty have also been reported for all three devices. Most complications requiring revision surgery were resolved by either fusion and/or disc replacement surgery. Interestingly, the causes of these complications seemed to be device-specific (i.e.; due to the design and/or make of the device).

For the ProDisc-L, the major complication described in the literature referred to the vertical split fracture of the vertebral body following total disc replacement. This occurrence was described by Shim et al in 2 separate cases that were not revised or treated surgically, but experienced prolonged back pain as a result[45]. An additional complication in the form of acquired spondylolysis was described by Schulte et al[46]. Authors attributed this complication to inaccurate implant size and positioning.

For the CHARITÉ Artificial Disc, the key complications were observed on the earlier devices, which were gamma sterilized in air and thus had a potential for oxidation of the core polyethylene nucleus [38]. Complications due to this oxidation process were described by Van Ooij et al (and Punt et al, as this paper reiterate data from the Van Ooij patient population)[41, 42]. This issue was resolved with a process change in 1998 to gamma sterilization in nitrogen. In a review of the RCT patient population, Geisler et al also evaluated the rate of neurological complications in the arthroplasty group vs. fusion group. The rate of neurological complication was described as exceedingly low in both groups with no statistically significant differences between groups.

While little has been published so far on the Maverick Total Disc Arthroplasty System, one article described an early removal of the Maverick Total Disc Arthroplasty System [47]. This removal was performed one year after implantation due to severe persistent back pain. Intraoperatively, gross metallosis around the articulation of the device was observed. The revision was successful and included a 360 degs fusion. Metallosis was thus cited as a potential complication for devices consisting of a metal-on-metal design. Zeh et al presented an additional potential complication: due to this metal-on-metal structure of the Maverick Total Disc Arthroplasty System, cobalt and chromium ions from the device were being released into the bloodstream [48]. In this study, cobalt and chromium ions from subjects implanted with the Maverick Total Disc Arthroplasty System were evaluated and compared to ion levels in total hip arthroplasty (THA) patients. Zeh et al found that concentrations of Cr/Co measured in the serum were similar in terms of their level to the values measured in THA metal-on-metal combinations or exceed those values reported in the literature. As a result, while Zeh et al did not recommend holding back with the implantation of the device, they did suggest long-term clinical evaluations to determine the clinical impact of high ion levels in serum and also recommended discussions with patients on the potential health effects of the prosthesis.

3.7 Special patient population analyses

The clinical outcomes for selective patient populations (e.g.; smokers, >60yr old) were discussed in multiple papers, more specifically for the ProDisc-L device. Bertagnoli et al lead these efforts with 4 publications presenting clinical data on arthroplasty with ProDisc-L in patients with: 1) single-level arthroplasty[15]; 2) multi-level arthroplasty[16]; 3) patients 60-years or older[49]; 4) smokers [50]; and 5) arthroplasty cases adjacent to a fused level [51]. While Bertagnoli et al repeatedly stated the importance of proper patient selection in each and every paper, all the results presented in these studies concluded that spinal arthroplasty with ProDisc-L successfully addressed low-back pain in these specific patient populations. Hannibal et al recently compared one- vs. two-level arthroplasty cases at the 2-year follow-up to try and establish whether one-level cases were experiencing greater clinical improvements as compared to the two-level cases. This hypothesis was not verified as differences in clinical improvements between one- and two-level cases were marginal [52]. Yaszay et al approached the problem from a different angle and evaluated patients outcomes based on a radiographic observation, i.e.; preoperative disc height [53]. Yaszay et al observed that patients with greater disc collapse experienced a greater benefit from total disc replacement, as compared to patients with less collapsed intervertebral discs. On average, patients in all of Bertagnoli et al and Yaszay et al series showed significant clinical improvement following arthroplasty.

Using the CHARITÉ Artificial Disc IDE RCT patient population, sub-analyses by patient types were also published by Guyer et al and Geisler et al. Specifically, patients were stratified by age at surgery (18-45 vs. 46-60) or whether they had had prior surgery or not[54, 55]. In both cases, there was no difference in clinical outcome between groups, whether patients were 18-45 or 46-60, or whether patient did or did not have prior surgery. Along the same trend, Geisler et al also evaluated the clinical outcomes of those patients from the CHARITÉ Artificial Disc RCT that did not improve with arthroplasty and needed revision surgery to a fusion. These patients (7.1% of all arthroplasty cases) did not improve, despite the revision surgery, further highlighting the importance of proper patient selection, and possibly, the fact that patient selection still remains a somewhat approximate science(59)[56].

3.8 Health economics evaluations

The impact of spinal arthroplasty on health care economics were reviewed for both the CHARITÉ Artificial Disc and the ProDisc-L. Guyer et al analyzed the costs related to a CHARITÉ Artificial Disc arthroplasty compared to: 1) an anterior fusion with autograft: 2) anterior fusion with rhBMP-2 (Infuse Bone Graft and LT-Cages) as well as 3) instrumented posterior lumbar interbody fusion. This analysis included the cost of revision surgery at the rate estimated in the published literature. Guyer et al concluded that all fusion procedures were more costly than the arthroscopy approach by 12.0% (ALIF with autograft) to 36.5% (ALIF with rhBMP-2 and posterior fusion)[57].

A similar analysis by Levin et al evaluated the costs of 1- and 2-level arthroplasty vs. 360 degs fusion. This study did not include possible needs for revisions. Nevertheless, one-level arthroplasty cases were found to be less costly than one-level fusions ($35,592 for arthroplasty vs. $46,280 for 360 deg fusion) while two-level cases were similar for both groups ($55,524 for arthroplasty vs. $56,823 for fusion)[58].

4. Discussion

From 2002 to 2008, a significant volume of data was made available on the clinical impact of arthroplasty. Sixty studies related to the clinical use of arthroplasty were published in peer-reviewed papers, of which 35 described data collected prospectively and 18 represented data from multi-center studies. The total number of patients described in the literature for spinal arthroplasty is difficult to evaluate, since many studies are early data releases or sub-analyses of the main randomized controlled trials performed for each new device. Thus, a given patient population might have been discussed in multiple papers. Overall, however, it was estimated that approximately 1,600 patients were included in the current literature.

The RCTs for the ProDisc-L and the CHARITÉ Artificial Disc both demonstrated the non-inferiority of the arthroplasty procedure, compared to their respective controls (ALIF for CHARITÉ Artificial Disc, 360 degs fusion for ProDisc-L. The complete RCT data for Maverick Total Disc Arthroplasty System and FlexiCore Intervertebral Disc are not yet published.) For some specific clinical outcomes such as pain, disability, and hospital stay, arthroplasty patients experienced greater clinical outcomes at some of the follow-up time points. For the CHARITÉ Artificial Disc RCT, arthroplasty patients fared statistically better than fusion on pain and disability for all but the 24-month follow-up time point. Hospital stay was also significantly shorter in the CHARITÉ Artificial Disc group as compared to the fusion group. As for ProDisc-L, pain scores were statistically better in the investigational cohort as compared to control. In addition, most other case series, for any of the given arthroplasty products, including those with short- and long-term follow-up data, presented favorable overall outcomes for spinal lumbar arthroplasty.

The issues of range of motion, heterotopic ossification, and sagittal balance have also drawn significant attention. While accurate and reproducible measurement of the lumbar ROM may be a significant limitation to collect meaningful data, average ROM at the 2-year time point throughout the studies evaluated herein were at ~ 7-10 degs. In addition, restoration of sagittal balance was observed for each device, the CHARITÉ Artificial Disc, the ProDisc-L as well as the Maverick Total Disc Arthroplasty System.

This review contained however somewhat contradictory data on the issue of facet and adjacent-level degeneration. While two of the 10year studies showed very small instances of facet and/or adjacent-level degeneration, others reported nearly a 1/3 of all cases with either CHARITÉ Artificial Disc or ProDisc-L developing changes in facet morphology. The inconsistency in these results points at potential surgeon-specific techniques and approaches that may impact the long-term benefits of both procedures.

Surgeon-specific variability in technique and proficiency was also cited in cases of revision. In fact, a study by Regan et al evaluating the occurrence of revision in low-volume vs. high-volume center, confirmed that surgeon in low-volume centers may incur greater peri-operative complications, however none that affected long-term outcomes[59]. Nevertheless, revisions were often found to be associated with technical errors, such as errors in positioning or sizing of the implant.

This critical importance of proper technique was in fact described in the 2 technique papers discussed herein. Both these publications stressed the importance of proper patient selection, a recurrent theme in almost all arthroplasty discussions.

Three types of major complications were described or foreseen in the current literature: 1) vertebral body split due to the ProDisc-L keel design; 2) oxidation of the core polymer nucleus, a problem specific to first generation CHARITÉ I prosthesis; and 3) metallosis and long-term impact of metal ions in the body. While the issue of metallosis and metal ions still needs to be thoroughly investigated, the problems related to vertebral body split only occurred once in the published literature, and as such, may represent a rare occurrence, and that of core oxidation, has been since resolved with new sterilization techniques following which core oxidation of the polymer nucleus is not observed. Thus, possible complications related to devices with metal-on-poly designs seem to be fairly limited.

Finally, low rates of complication and adverse event were observed for most of all analyzed patients. For the ProDisc-L, smokers as well as patients 60 years of age seemed to experience similar benefit from the procedure. In all these studies, however, authors reiterated the importance of proper patient selection, thus concluding that, while all analyzed patient types experienced clinical benefit from the procedure, specific care must be given to only operate on appropriate patients.

Finally, no technology is sustainable in today's market place if its cost is prohibitive. Thus, the impact of arthroplasty on health economics was also investigated. Both, the CHARITÉ Artificial Disc and the ProDisc-L study came up at a lower cost than their fusion controls, whether potential revision costs were included or not. No data on cost exists yet for the Maverick Total Disc Arthroplasty System and the FlexiCore Intervertebral Disc.

5. TDR surgery

The typical diseased lumbar segment considered for artificial disc technologies at L4-L5 or L5-S1 has advanced degenerative disc disease with loss of vertical height and lordosis, dehydration changes, adjacent Modic endplate changes, and little motion on dynamic studies (see Figure 1). The natural progression of degenerative disease disc limits the joint mobility and this biomechanical fact places more forces on the adjacent levels then in the normal situation. The artificial lumbar disc, by restoring normal motion, height, and lordosis, will decrease the forces on the adjacent levels. Thus, theoretically, levels adjacent to a dynamically stabilized level may have beneficial effects compared to the natural history of the unoperated degenerative state. Clearly some patients will benefit from the decreased force on the adjacent vertebral level(s) following a dynamic stabilization (arthroplasty) compared to a static stabilization (fusion). Estimates of the rate and groups of patients at maximum benefit will need to await long-term clinical follow up studies with lumbar arthroplasty devices similar to the hip and knee arthroplasty registries. Also, although a dynamically stabilized level can be converted to a fusion, a fused level cannot be converted to a dynamic joint. Thus, artificial technology can be thought of as a definitive procedure for the vast majority of patients that can be converted to a fusion if the pain and functional goals are not met or degenerative changes occur in the posterior elements and the arthrodesis level is believed to be the pain generator.

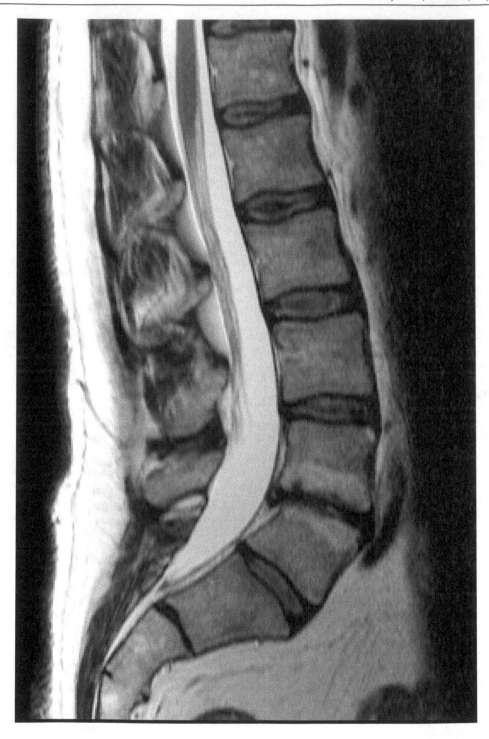

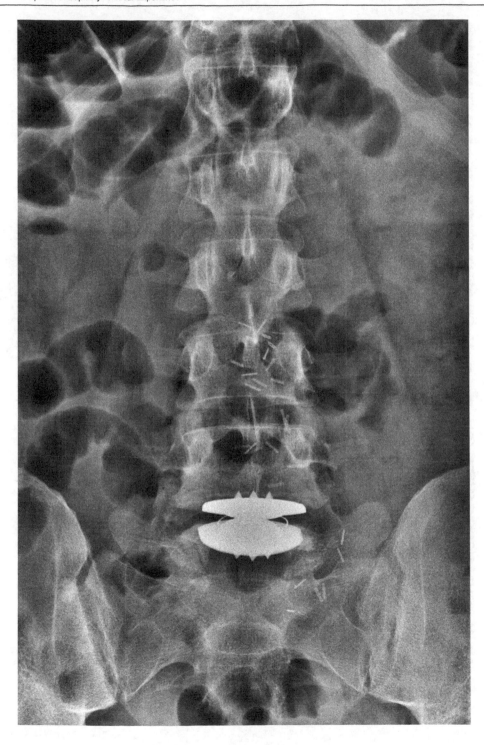

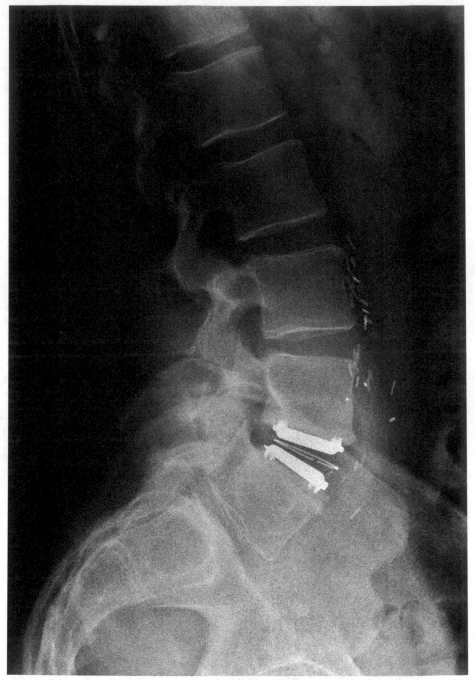

Fig. 1. Typical radiographies for a TDR patient. 1a. Pre-operative MRI. 1b. Post-operative A-P radiography. 1c. Post-operative lateral radiography.

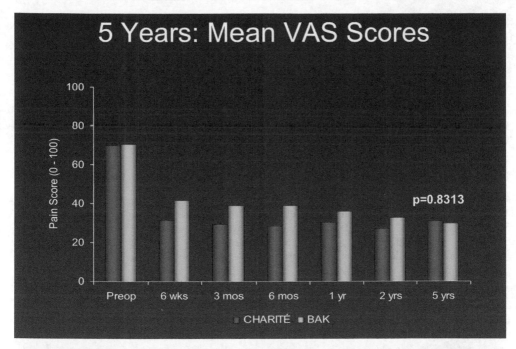

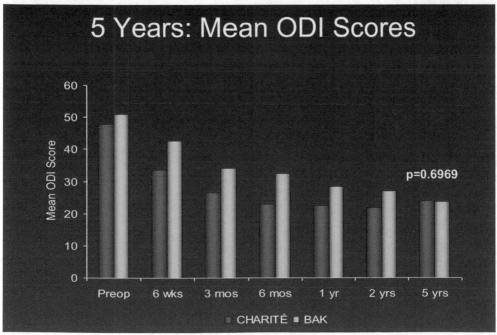

Fig. 2. Five years results from the Charité FDA IDE prospective randomized study. 2a. ODI. 2b. VAS.

6. Revision techniques

If a CHARITÉ artificial disc were required to be revised, there would be two options available. One approach would be anterior reoperation. This would involve dissecting the retroperitoneal area and dealing with the post-op scarring and hence increased risk of great vessel damage, ureteral damage, and damage to the sympathetic nerves compared to a case without prior dissection and scarring in the retroperitoneal space. A revision allows removal, position adjustment or size change of the CHARITÉ artificial disc. The plastic core would be removed first, and then the metal endplates are separated from the bony endplates by using a chisel between them and levering away from the bone into the disc space. This would allow the placement of another artificial disc in the disc space or the conversion to a fusion. Alternately, a posterior operation with rod-screw stabilization and posterior lateral fusion could be used to fuse the lumbar segment, which would use the CHARITÉ artificial disc as an anterior load share device. As with all surgical decision making, understanding the biomechanical reasoning and etiology of clinical failure is of the utmost importance. In patients with recurring or persistent pain the characterization of the pain generator is often more important than the exact surgical technique used. Radiologic studies such as dynamic A-P and Lat x-ray and multislice CT will aid in understanding failure of the device or progression of the degenerative anatomic changes. Radiologic and provocative studies, including discography, anesthetic or negative discography, nerve root blocks, epidural injections, and facet injections may all be utilized to identify the anatomic site of the pain generator.

7. Long-term follow-up of TDR patients

The initial CHARITÉ was planned with a 2-year follow-up period. At the request of the FDA the follow-up period was extended to 5-years and the sites requested to participate in the "new" 2 to 5 year follow-up period. Multiple sites did participate in this extended reporting period and formed the basis of the 5-year CHARITÉ results. The CHARITÉ 5-year ODI and VAS results (Figure 2a and 2b respectively) were substantially the same as the 2-years follow-up results[60]. Despite the prospective collection of the these results, critics formulated objections to these reported good results[61].

8. Conclusion

Overall, there were only minor differences between devices in terms of overall clinical and radiographic outcome. Significant improvements in clinical outcomes were seen with all evaluated devices, regardless of make or design. An average maintenance of motion post-operatively was described, along with relatively low rates of revision. Differences between devices were mostly apparent in complication types: one potential complication for devices with keels was vertebral body split, while devices with metal-on-metal designs could cause metallosis and ion release in the serum. As for metal-on-poly devices, degradation of the polymer core was also mentioned as a potential complication, albeit one that is not relevant for the current metal-on-poly devices. Specific emphasis was found in most of all publications on proper technique and patient selection, regardless of implant design. Finally, arthroplasty was found to be less costly than fusion.

9. References

[1] Griffith SL, Shelokov AP, Buttner-Janz K, LeMaire JP, Zeegers WS. A multicenter retrospective study of the clinical results of the LINK SB Charite intervertebral

prosthesis. The initial European experience. *Spine.* Aug 15 1994;19(16):1842-1849.

[2] Zigler J, Delamarter R, Spivak JM, et al. Results of the prospective, randomized, multicenter Food and Drug Administration investigational device exemption study of the ProDisc-L total disc replacement versus circumferential fusion for the treatment of 1-level degenerative disc disease. *Spine (Phila Pa 1976).* May 15 2007;32(11):1155-1162; discussion 1163.

[3] McAfee PC, Fedder IL, Saiedy S, Shucosky EM, Cunningham BW. SB Charite disc replacement: report of 60 prospective randomized cases in a US center. *J Spinal Disord Tech.* Aug 2003;16(4):424-433.

[4] Lemaire JP, Carrier H, Sari Ali E, Skalli W, Lavaste F. Clinical and Radiological Outcomes With the CHARITÉ™ Artificial Disc: A 10-Year Minimum Follow-Up. *J Spinal Disord.* 2005;18(4):353-359.

[5] Guyer RD, McAfee PC, Hochschuler SH, et al. Prospective randomized study of the Charite artificial disc: data from two investigational centers. *Spine J.* Nov-Dec 2004;4(6 Suppl):252S-259S.

[6] Geisler FH, Blumenthal SL, Guyer RD, et al. Neurological complications of lumbar artificial disc replacement and comparison of clinical results with those related to lumbar arthrodesis in the literature: results of a multicenter, prospective, randomized investigational device exemption study of Charite intervertebral disc. Invited submission from the Joint Section Meeting on Disorders of the Spine and Peripheral Nerves, March 2004. *J Neurosurg Spine.* Sep 2004;1(2):143-154.

[7] Blumenthal SL, McAfee PC, Guyer RD, et al. A Prospective, Randomized, Multicenter Food and Drug Administration Investigational Device Exemptions Study of Lumbar Total Disc Replacement with the CHARITÉ™ Artificial Disc Versus Lumbar Fusion Part I: Evaluation of Clinical Outcomes. *Spine.* 2005;30(14):1565-1575.

[8] McAfee PC, Cunningham B, Holsapple GA, et al. A Prospective, Randomized, Multicenter Food and Drug Administration Investigational Device Exemptions Study of Lumbar Total Disc Replacement with the CHARITÉ™ Artificial Disc Versus Lumbar Fusion Part II: Evaluation of Radiographic Outcomes and Correlation of Surgical Technique Accuracy with Clinical Outcomes. *Spine.* 2005;30(14):1576-1583.

[9] David T. Long-term results of one-level lumbar arthroplasty: minimum 10-year follow-up of the CHARITE artificial disc in 106 patients. *Spine (Phila Pa 1976).* Mar 15 2007;32(6):661-666.

[10] Ross R, Mirza AH, Norris HE, Khatri M. Survival and clinical outcome of SB Charite III disc replacement for back pain. *J Bone Joint Surg Br.* Jun 2007;89(6):785-789.

[11] Guyer RD, Blumenthal SL. Survival and clinical outcome of SB Charite III disc replacement for back pain. *J Bone Joint Surg Br.* Dec 2007;89(12):1673; author reply 1673-1674.

[12] Scott-Young MN. Survival and clinical outcome of SB Charite III disc replacement for back pain. *J Bone Joint Surg Br.* Dec 2007;89(12):1674; author reply 1674-1675.

[13] Bertagnoli R, Kumar S. Indications for full prosthetic disc arthroplasty: a correlation of clinical outcome against a variety of indications. *Eur Spine J.* Oct 2002;11 Suppl 2:S131-136.

[14] Tropiano P, Huang RC, Girardi FP, Cammisa FP, Jr., Marnay T. Lumbar total disc replacement. Seven to eleven-year follow-up. *J Bone Joint Surg Am.* Mar 2005;87(3):490-496.

[15] Bertagnoli R, Yue JJ, Shah RV, et al. The treatment of disabling single-level lumbar discogenic low back pain with total disc arthroplasty utilizing the Prodisc prosthesis: a prospective study with 2-year minimum follow-up. *Spine (Phila Pa 1976).* Oct 1 2005;30(19):2230-2236.

[16] Bertagnoli R, Yue JJ, Shah RV, et al. The treatment of disabling multilevel lumbar discogenic low back pain with total disc arthroplasty utilizing the ProDisc prosthesis: a prospective study with 2-year minimum follow-up. *Spine (Phila Pa 1976).* Oct 1 2005;30(19):2192-2199.

[17] Chung SS, Lee CS, Kang CS. Lumbar total disc replacement using ProDisc II: a prospective study with a 2-year minimum follow-up. *J Spinal Disord Tech.* Aug 2006;19(6):411-415.

[18] Delamarter RB, Fribourg DM, Kanim LE, Bae H. ProDisc artificial total lumbar disc replacement: introduction and early results from the United States clinical trial. *Spine (Phila Pa 1976).* Oct 15 2003;28(20):S167-175.

[19] Tropiano P, Huang RC, Girardi FP, Marnay T. Lumbar disc replacement: preliminary results with ProDisc II after a minimum follow-up period of 1 year. *J Spinal Disord Tech.* Aug 2003;16(4):362-368.

[20] Zigler JE, Burd TA, Vialle EN, Sachs BL, Rashbaum RF, Ohnmeiss DD. Lumbar spine arthroplasty: early results using the ProDisc II: a prospective randomized trial of arthroplasty versus fusion. *J Spinal Disord Tech.* Aug 2003;16(4):352-361.

[21] Zigler JE. Lumbar spine arthroplasty using the ProDisc II. *Spine J.* Nov-Dec 2004;4(6 Suppl):260S-267S.

[22] Fairbank JC, Pynsent PB. The Oswestry Disability Index. *Spine (Phila Pa 1976).* Nov 15 2000;25(22):2940-2952; discussion 2952.

[23] Fairbank JC. Use and abuse of Oswestry Disability Index. *Spine (Phila Pa 1976).* Dec 1 2007;32(25):2787-2789.

[24] Le Huec JC, Mathews H, Basso Y, et al. Clinical results of Maverick lumbar total disc replacement: two-year prospective follow-up. *Orthop Clin North Am.* Jul 2005;36(3):315-322.

[25] Le Huec JC, Basso Y, Aunoble S, Friesem T, Bruno MB. Influence of facet and posterior muscle degeneration on clinical results of lumbar total disc replacement: two-year follow-up. *J Spinal Disord Tech.* Jun 2005;18(3):219-223.

[26] Sasso RC, Foulk DM, Hahn M. Prospective, randomized trial of metal-on-metal artificial lumbar disc replacement: initial results for treatment of discogenic pain. *Spine (Phila Pa 1976).* Jan 15 2008;33(2):123-131.

[27] Cunningham BW, McAfee PC, Geisler FH, et al. Distribution of in vivo and in vitro range of motion following 1-level arthroplasty with the CHARITE artificial disc compared with fusion. *J Neurosurg Spine.* Jan 2008;8(1):7-12.

[28] Lim MR, Girardi FP, Zhang K, Huang RC, Peterson MG, Cammisa FP, Jr. Measurement of total disc replacement radiographic range of motion: a comparison of two techniques. *J Spinal Disord Tech.* Jun 2005;18(3):252-256.

[29] Lim MR, Loder RT, Huang RC, et al. Measurement error of lumbar total disc replacement range of motion. *Spine (Phila Pa 1976).* May 1 2006;31(10):E291-297.

[30] Huang RC, Girardi FP, Cammisa Jr FP, Tropiano P, Marnay T. Long-term flexion-extension range of motion of the prodisc total disc replacement. *J Spinal Disord Tech.* Oct 2003;16(5):435-440.

[31] Chung SS, Lee CS, Kang CS, Kim SH. The effect of lumbar total disc replacement on the spinopelvic alignment and range of motion of the lumbar spine. *J Spinal Disord Tech.* Jul 2006;19(5):307-311.

[32] Le Huec J, Basso Y, Mathews H, et al. The effect of single-level, total disc arthroplasty on sagittal balance parameters: a prospective study. *Eur Spine J.* Jun 2005;14(5):480-486.

[33] Tournier C, Aunoble S, Le Huec JC, et al. Total disc arthroplasty: consequences for sagittal balance and lumbar spine movement. *Eur Spine J.* Mar 2007;16(3):411-421.

[34] McAfee PC, Cunningham BW, Devine J, Williams E, Yu-Yahiro J. Classification of heterotopic ossification (HO) in artificial disk replacement. *J Spinal Disord Tech.* Aug 2003;16(4):384-389.

[35] Tortolani PJ, Cunningham BW, Eng M, McAfee PC, Holsapple GA, Adams KA. Prevalence of heterotopic ossification following total disc replacement. A prospective, randomized study of two hundred and seventy-six patients. *J Bone Joint Surg Am.* Jan 2007;89(1):82-88.

[36] Huang RC, Tropiano P, Marnay T, Girardi FP, Lim MR, Cammisa FP, Jr. Range of motion and adjacent level degeneration after lumbar total disc replacement. *Spine J.* May-Jun 2006;6(3):242-247.

[37] Trouillier H, Kern P, Refior HJ, Muller-Gerbl M. A prospective morphological study of facet joint integrity following intervertebral disc replacement with the CHARITE Artificial Disc. *Eur Spine J.* Feb 2006;15(2):174-182.

[38] David T. Revision of a Charite artificial disc 9.5 years in vivo to a new Charite artificial disc: case report and explant analysis. *Eur Spine J.* Jun 2005;14(5):507-511.

[39] Leary SP, Regan JJ, Lanman TH, Wagner WH. Revision and explantation strategies involving the CHARITE lumbar artificial disc replacement. *Spine (Phila Pa 1976).* Apr 20 2007;32(9):1001-1011.

[40] McAfee PC, Geisler FH, Saiedy S, et al. Revisability of the CHARITÉ Artificial Disc Replacement - Analysis of 688 Patients Enrolled in the U.S. IDE Study of the CHARITÉ Artificial Disc. *Spine.* 2006 2006;31(11):1217-1226.

[41] Punt IM, Visser VM, van Rhijn LW, et al. Complications and reoperations of the SB Charite lumbar disc prosthesis: experience in 75 patients. *Eur Spine J.* Jan 2008;17(1):36-43.

[42] van Ooij A, Oner FC, Verbout AJ. Complications of artificial disc replacement: a report of 27 patients with the SB Charite disc. *J Spinal Disord Tech.* Aug 2003;16(4):369-383.

[43] Geisler FH. Surgical Technique of Lumbar Artificial Disc Replacement with the CHARITE™ Artificial Disc. *Neurosurgery.* 2005;56:ONS46-57.

[44] Gumbs AA, Shah RV, Yue JJ, Sumpio B. The open anterior paramedian retroperitoneal approach for spine procedures. *Arch Surg.* Apr 2005;140(4):339-343.

[45] Shim CS, Lee S, Maeng DH, Lee SH. Vertical split fracture of the vertebral body following total disc replacement using ProDisc: report of two cases. *J Spinal Disord Tech.* Oct 2005;18(5):465-469.

[46] Schulte TL, Lerner T, Hackenberg L, Liljenqvist U, Bullmann V. Acquired spondylolysis after implantation of a lumbar ProDisc II prosthesis: case report and review of the literature. *Spine (Phila Pa 1976).* Oct 15 2007;32(22):E645-648.

[47] Francois J, Coessens R, Lauweryns P. Early removal of a Maverick disc prosthesis: surgical findings and morphological changes. *Acta Orthop Belg*. Feb 2007;73(1):122-127.

[48] Zeh A, Planert M, Siegert G, Lattke P, Held A, Hein W. Release of cobalt and chromium ions into the serum following implantation of the metal-on-metal Maverick-type artificial lumbar disc (Medtronic Sofamor Danek). *Spine (Phila Pa 1976)*. Feb 1 2007;32(3):348-352.

[49] Bertagnoli R, Yue JJ, Nanieva R, et al. Lumbar total disc arthroplasty in patients older than 60 years of age: a prospective study of the ProDisc prosthesis with 2-year minimum follow-up period. *J Neurosurg Spine*. Feb 2006;4(2):85-90.

[50] Bertagnoli R, Yue JJ, Kershaw T, et al. Lumbar total disc arthroplasty utilizing the ProDisc prosthesis in smokers versus nonsmokers: a prospective study with 2-year minimum follow-up. *Spine (Phila Pa 1976)*. Apr 20 2006;31(9):992-997.

[51] Bertagnoli R, Yue JJ, Fenk-Mayer A, Eerulkar J, Emerson JW. Treatment of symptomatic adjacent-segment degeneration after lumbar fusion with total disc arthroplasty by using the prodisc prosthesis: a prospective study with 2-year minimum follow up. *J Neurosurg Spine*. Feb 2006;4(2):91-97.

[52] Hannibal M, Thomas DJ, Low J, Hsu KY, Zucherman J. ProDisc-L total disc replacement: a comparison of 1-level versus 2-level arthroplasty patients with a minimum 2-year follow-up. *Spine (Phila Pa 1976)*. Oct 1 2007;32(21):2322-2326.

[53]Yaszay B, Bendo JA, Goldstein JA, Quirno M, Spivak JM, Errico TJ. Effect of intervertebral disc height on postoperative motion and outcomes after ProDisc-L lumbar disc replacement. *Spine (Phila Pa 1976)*. Mar 1 2008;33(5):508-512; discussion 513.

[54] Guyer RD, Geisler FH, Blumenthal SL, McAfee PC, Mullin BB. Effect of age on clinical and radiographic outcomes and adverse events following 1-level lumbar arthroplasty after a minimum 2-year follow-up. *J Neurosurg Spine*. Feb 2008;8(2):101-107.

[55] Geisler FH, Guyer RD, Blumenthal SL, et al. Effect of previous surgery on clinical outcome following 1-level lumbar arthroplasty. *J Neurosurg Spine*. Feb 2008;8(2):108-114.

[56] Geisler FH, Guyer RD, Blumenthal SL, et al. Patient selection for lumbar arthroplasty and arthrodesis: the effect of revision surgery in a controlled, multicenter, randomized study. *J Neurosurg Spine*. Jan 2008;8(1):13-16.

[57] Guyer RD, Tromanhauser SG, Regan JJ. An economic model of one-level lumbar arthroplasty versus fusion. *Spine J*. Sep-Oct 2007;7(5):558-562.

[58] Levin DA, Bendo JA, Quirno M, Errico T, Goldstein J, Spivak J. Comparative charge analysis of one- and two-level lumbar total disc arthroplasty versus circumferential lumbar fusion. *Spine (Phila Pa 1976)*. Dec 1 2007;32(25):2905-2909.

[59] Regan JJ, McAfee PC, Blumenthal SL, et al. Evaluation of Surgical Volume and the Early Experience with Lumbar Total Disc Replacement as Part of the IDE Study of the CHARITÉ™ Artificial Disc. *Spine*. Sept 1, 2006 2006;31(19):2270-2276.

[60] Guyer RD, McAfee PC, Banco RJ, et al. Prospective, randomized, multicenter Food and Drug Administration investigational device exemption study of lumbar total disc replacement with the CHARITE artificial disc versus lumbar fusion: five-year follow-up. *Spine J*. May 2009;9(5):374-386.

[61] van den Eerenbeemt KD, Ostelo RW, van Royen BJ, Peul WC, van Tulder MW. Total disc replacement surgery for symptomatic degenerative lumbar disc disease: a systematic review of the literature. *Eur Spine J*. Aug 2010;19(8):1262-1280.

6

Cervical Disc Arthroplasty

Bruce V. Darden

OrthoCarolina Spine Center, Charlotte

USA

1. Introduction

For more than 50 years, anterior cervical discectomy and fusion (ACDF) has been the workhorse procedure for cervical degenerative pathology. (Bailey & Badgely, 1960; Cloward, 1961; Robinson & Smith, 1955)   The procedure has yielded successful results clinically in multiple large series. (Bohlman et al, 1993; Gore & Sepic, 1984)   Advances in allograft and cage techniques as well as the use of anterior plating systems have diminished complications in ACDF. However, concerns about adjacent segment degeneration (ASD) have tempered some enthusiasm for the procedure. Gore et al (Gore & Sepic, 1998) reviewed a series of 50 ACDF patients followed long term. Almost universally, the patients developed ASD. One-third of the cohort developed recurrent pain with half of the symptomatic group requiring additional surgery. Hilibrand et al (Hilibrand et al, 1999) evaluated a group of 374 patients undergoing ACDF. They showed a 2.9% per year risk of development of symptomatic ASD, with two thirds of the symptomatic patients requiring additional surgery. Goffin et al (Goffin et al, 1995) prospectively followed a series of ACDF patients who underwent the procedure for either a degenerative or traumatic condition. Follow-up was for five to nine years. Sixty percent of the patients developed ASD, equally distributed between the older degenerative population and the younger traumatic population, providing evidence that fusion may accelerate degenerative changes. Goffin et al (Goffin et al, 2004) reviewed a larger series of ACDF patients followed for an average of 8.3 years. In this group, 92% of the patients developed ASD, though they had a much lower rate of additional surgical procedures, 6.1% for the entire length of follow-up, distinctly lower than Hilibrand et al. Numerous cadaveric biomechanical studies (Eck et al, 2002; Pospiech et al, 1999) evaluating adjacent level intradiscal pressures and range of motion in simulated fusion models have shown that both increase after fusion. These altered biomechanics may thus accelerate ASD.

Against this background, centers began experimenting with cervical disc arthroplasty in the 1980s. Cummins and collaborators at the Frenchay Hospital, Bristol, England developed a metal-on-metal ball and socket arthroplasty and implanted it on a small series of patients in the 1990s. (Cummins et al, 1998) The arthroplasty underwent a number of design changes and is now known as Prestige. Bryan, in the US, developed a one piece metal-on-polymer device called the Bryan Cervical Disc Replacement, initially evaluated clinically in Europe. (Goffin et al, 2002) ProDisc-C arthroplasty is a metal-on-polyethylene implant adopted from the ProDisc-L lumbar disc arthroplasty developed by Thierry Marnay. (Delamarter & Pradhan, 2004) Since these first three devices have been developed, the number of cervical disc arthroplasties has proliferated. The literature in this nascent field is limited, but growing each year.

2. Types of cervical disc arthroplasty

It is beyond the scope of this chapter to catalogue all of the cervical disc arthroplasties available; the devices with the most clinical experience will be discussed.

2.1 Prestige
The technology from the early designs of Cummins et al was acquired by Medtronic Sofamor Danek (Memphis, Tennessee) and rebadged Prestige. With Prestige I, the initial ball and socket design which was entirely fabricated from stainless steel, was converted to a ball and trough design, allowing limited translation. The anterior flanges were diminished in size and a locking screw added to prevent bone screw backout. Prestige II was further modified by again reducing the anterior flange and modifying the endplates to allow bone ingrowth. Prestige ST was the design evaluated in the United States as part of the Food and Drug Administration (FDA) investigational device evaluational (IDE) study. This arthroplasty incorporates the features of Prestige II with further shortened anterior flanges. The final design is Prestige LP, a major change from its predecessors. Instead of stainless steel, the Prestige LP is made from a titanium ceramic composite, preserving the ball and trough bearing design. It has a titanium plasma spray on the endplates for bone ingrowth, as well as two pairs of rails allowing immediate fixation. The flange and locking bone screws have been removed. The Prestige LP, being made of titanium, has a better compatibility than stainless steel in MRI imaging. (Figure 1)

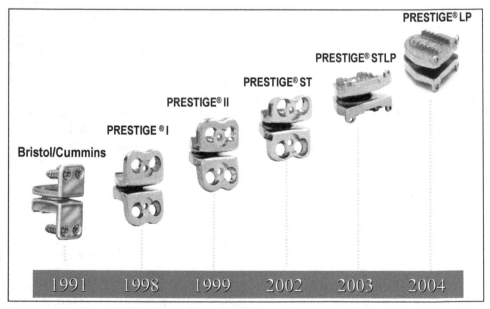

(Courtesy of Medtronic Sofamor Danek, Memphis, Tennessee)

Fig. 1. Prestige Cervical Disc evolution

2.2 Bryan Cervical Disc Prosthesis

Bryan Cervical Disc Prosthesis (Medtronic Sofamor Danek, Memphis, Tennessee) consists of a nucleus made of polyurethane between two titanium alloy endplates in a clamshell configuration. (Figure 2) There are two bearing surfaces in the arthroplasty at the interfaces between the nucleus and the endplates. A polyurethane sheath attaches to the endplates and surrounds the nucleus. Sterile saline is injected between the outer sheath and the nucleus as lubricant. The endplates have a titanium porous coating for bone ingrowth and a small flange anteriorly to prevent posterior migration.

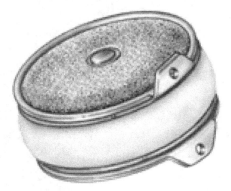

(Courtesy of Medtronic Sofamor Danek, Memphis, Tennessee)

Fig. 2. Bryan Cervical Disc Prosthesis

2.3 ProDisc-C

ProDisc-C Cervical Disc Prosthesis (Synthes, West Chester, Pennsylvania) has a ball and socket design, with endplates made of a cobalt-chrome alloy. The endplates have keels for immediate fixation and titanium plasma spray backing for bone ingrowth. The bearing surface has an articulating dome of ultra high molecular weight polyethylene (UHMWPE) attached to the inferior endplate and a concave polished socket integral to the superior endplate. (Figure 3)

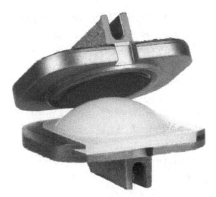

(Courtesy of Synthes, West Chester, Pennsylvania)

Fig. 3. ProDisc-C Cervical Disc

2.4 Porous-Coated Motion (PCM) Cervical Arthroplasty

The Porous-Coated Motion (PCM) Cervical Arthroplasty (Cervitech, Rockaway, New Jersey) consists of two cobalt-chrome-molybdenum (CoCrMo) endplates that have a titanium calcium phosphate porous coated backing for bone ingrowth. The device is inserted by a "press-fit" method, but the endplates have transverse serrated rows of teeth that resist migration. The bearing surface is an ultra high molecular weight polyethylene (UHMWPE) convex insert of large radius of curvature attached to the inferior endplate which articulates with the polished CoCrMo concave surface of the superior endplate. (Figure 4)

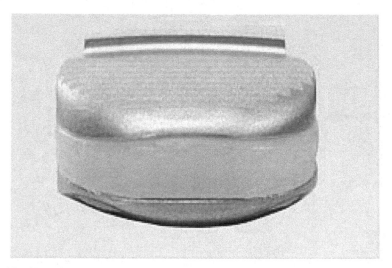

(Courtesy of Paul McAfee, MD)

Fig. 4. Porous Coated Motion (PCM) Cervical Arthroplasty

3. Biomechanics

Cervical disc arthroplasty attempts to replicate the normal kinematics of the subaxial cervical spine, defined as the segments from C3 to C7. The subaxial cervical spine contributes 60% of the flexion/extension motion of the cervical spine with each segment accounting for between 14 to 22 degrees of motion (Dvorak et al, 1993; Dvorak et al, 1991; Penning, 1978). The flexion/extension arc, together with translational movements due to slight relative facet motion, results in coupled motions. Coupled motions also occur with lateral bending and thus axial rotation. These coupled motions result in differences in the center of rotation of each motion segment. Since the center of rotation is not fixed, there are instantaneous centers of rotation. (ICR) Penning (Penning, 1978) established normalized ICR for each segment, which were further defined by Amevo et al (Amevo et al, 1991) The normalized ICR for each segment are shown in figure 5 (Bogduk & Mercer, 2000) and are grossly posterior and inferior to the center of the caudal vertebral endplate. Arthroplasty designs with a ball and socket articulation have a predetermined center of rotation (ie: ProDisc-C). These more constrained designs have to be implanted more precisely to match the physiologic center of rotation to avoid increased strain on the facet joints. (Darden & Raposo, pending)

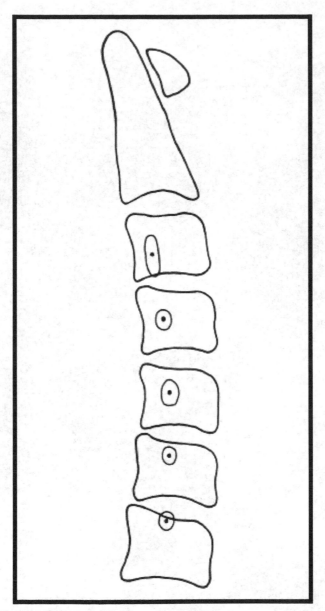

(Reprinted from: Bogduk N, Mercer S. Clin Biomechanics, 2000)

Fig. 5. Mean instantaneous axes of rotation for each motion segment of the cervical spine depicted with a dot. Two standard deviation range of distribution is located within the enclosed circles shown.

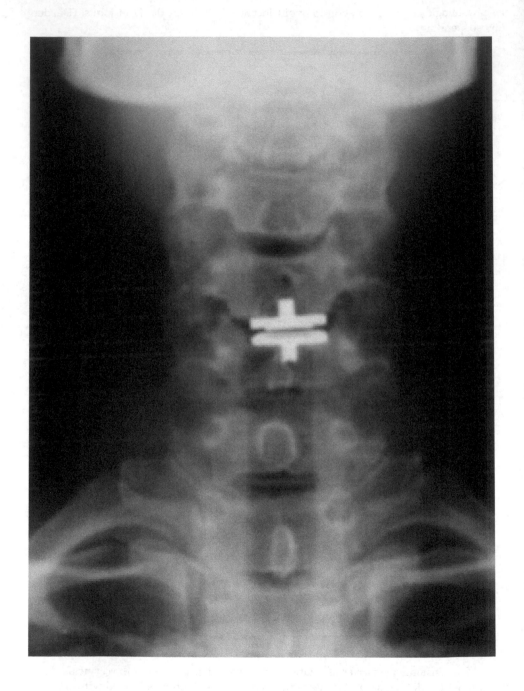

Fig. 6-A.

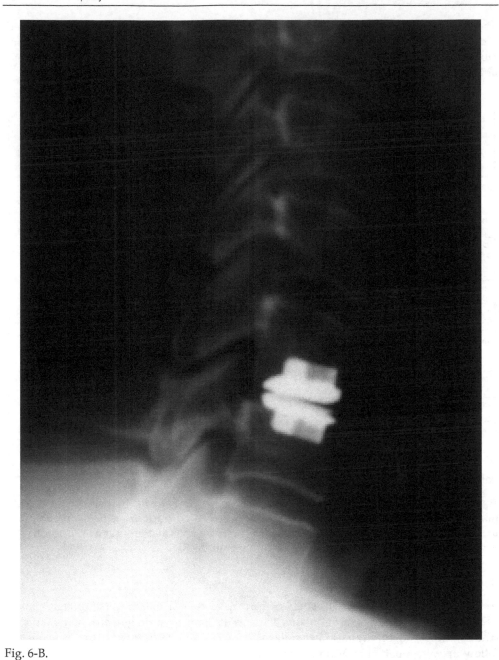

Fig. 6-B.

Fig. 6-A, B. AP and lateral radiographs of ProDisc-C

In the cervical spine, the dominant plane of motion is sagittal. Constraint is therefore defined as limitation of anterior-posterior translational motion. (Huang et al, 2003)   An unconstrained arthroplasty would allow unrestricted motion while a fully constrained arthroplasty would allow only flexion/extension without any anterior-posterior translation. However, compared to large joints, the differences in constraint in cervical disc arthroplasties are limited. (Darden & Raposo, pending) (Table 1)

Implant	Bryan®	Prestige ST®	Prodisc-C®	PCM-V®
Manufacturer	Medtronic Sofamor Danek,	Medtronic Sofamor Danek	Synthes	Cervitech
Bearing surface materials	Metal-on-poly; Titanium end plates, polycarbonate urethane nucleus	Metal-on-metal; Stainless steel	Metal-on-poly; Chrome cobalt, UHMWPE	Metal-on-poly; chrome cobalt, UHMWPE
Bearing surface geometry	Biconvex nucleus articulating with upper and lower endplates	Ball and trough design	Ball and socket design	Ball and socket design (shallow sphere)
Primary (immediate) fixation	Milling technique creates concave endplate surfaces to fit convex endplates of the device.	Anterior flanges with screws	Keels	LP: Press-fit, ridges
Degree of constraint	Unconstrained	Semi-constrained	Semi-constrained	Semi-constrained
Relative constraint	Least	Less	Most	Less
Implant center or rotation	Variable; lies at center of the mobile nucleus	Variable; superior to disc space	Fixed; inferior to disc space	Variable; inferior to disc space

Table 1. Summary of implant features and design characteristics.

A number of arthroplasties have been evaluated biomechanically versus simulated fusion in human cadaveric models. These routinely show increased adjacent segment motion and increased adjacent segment disc pressures in the fusion simulations compared to cervical disc arthroplasty. (DiAngelo et al, 2003; Dmitriev et al, 2005)

4. Clinical results

As a result of the US FDA IDE studies, there have been a number of thorough clinical evaluations of cervical disc arthroplasty. These trials have been designed as non-inferiority studies, comparing cervical disc arthroplasty to ACDF. The Prestige ST results at two years follow-up were reported by Mummaneni et al. (Mummaneni et al, 2007) The study, similar to all of the FDA IDE studies, was a prospective, randomized, multicenter trial comparing Prestige ST cervical disc arthroplasty to ACDF for one level pathology. Five hundred forty-one patients were enrolled with 1:1 randomization; over 75% of patients were available for two-year follow-up. There were no statistically significant differences in the revision surgeries at the index level (3.4% ACDF, 1.9% Prestige ST). However, the rate of surgery at adjacent levels was statistically higher for ACDF (3.4% versus 1.1%, p=0.0492). Neurological success, defined as maintenance or improvement in the neurological exam, was better with Prestige ST (92.8%) than ACDF (84.3%). Clinically, the patients were evaluated by Short-form 36 (SF-36), Visual Analogue Scale (VAS) and the Neck Disability Index (NDI). While both groups improved significantly from the preoperative state, there was no statistically significant difference between the groups at final follow-up. Overall success was defined as an NDI improvement ≥ 15 points, maintenance of the neurological status and the absence of implant-related adverse events. The arthroplasty group showed overall success in 79.3% of the patients compared to 67.8% in the ACDF group. As a sidebar, the Prestige ST patients were able to return to work on average at 45 days postoperatively, compared to 61 days for the ACDF patients.

A small prospective study compared results for Prestige LP and ACDF at a minimum of two years follow-up. Single and multilevel procedures were evaluated by VAS, NDI, SF-36 and Japanese Orthopedic Association scores. Clinically, while both groups improved significantly, there was no statistical difference between them. Motion was preserved in the Prestige LP group at a mean of 13.9° on flexion/extension lateral radiographs of two years. (Peng et al, 2011)

For the Bryan Cervical Disc Replacement, Goffin et al reported on the European experience, a multicenter, prospective, nonrandomized study, including both single-level and multi-level implants. Ninety-eight patients were evaluated at the 4 to 6 year follow-up point, 89 single-level patients and 9 two-level patients. The patients maintained improvement clinically at all evaluation periods. Approximately 90% of the patients had good or excellent results by Odum's criteria. The success rate for the arthroplasties, estimated by Kaplan-Meier analysis was 94% at 7 years postoperatively. One patient had removal of the arthroplasty for progressive spinal cord compression due to posterior osteophytes. (Goffin et al, 2010)

The Bryan FDA IDE study results at two years were published by Heller et al (Heller et al, 2009). Four hundred sixty-three patients enrolled, with 242 having a single-level Bryan Cervical Disc Replacement and 221 having single-level ACDF. The Bryan patients had statistically significantly improved NDI and VAS scores compared to the ACDF group at two years follow-up. Other clinical parameters improved equally between the two groups. Overall success at final follow-up was better in the Bryan patients (82.6%) versus the ACDF controls (72.7%), (p=0.010). As with the Prestige IDE patients, the Bryan patients returned to work sooner than did the ACDF patients.

Riew et al (Riew et al, 2008) evaluated a subset of patients enrolled in the Prestige ST or Bryan IDE studies that were determined to have a cervical myelopathy, defined as being hyperreflexic, having clonus or having a Nurick grade ≥ 1. In most of the patients, the cause of the myelopathy was a disc herniation. Because of enrollment criteria, multilevel cervical disease or patients with ossification of the posterior longitudinal ligament (OPLL) were excluded. A total of 107 patients in both studies were deemed myelopathic and underwent cervical disc arthroplasty. Compared to the ACDF patients, arthroplasty patients with myelopathy showed similar clinical improvement. There were no arthroplasty patients who deteriorated neurologically, suggesting that myelopathy confined to a single disc level without OPLL or retrovertebral osteophytes can be treated successfully with cervical disc arthroplasty.

Murrey et al (Murrey et al, 2009) published the two year ProDisc-C IDE study. The study was structured similarly to the Prestige ST and Bryan studies, with 209 patients enrolled, 103 who underwent ProDisc-C arthroplasty and 106 who had an ACDF. Both groups showed improvement by all clinical after parameters; NDI, SF-36, VAS arm and neck pain scores and neurological success. A significant difference was in the rate of re-operation: 8.5% in the ACDF group versus 1.8% in the ProDisc-C group (p= 0.033).

Delamarter et al further evaluated the ProDisc-C IDE patients as well as 136 patients who received ProDisc-C in the continued access phase of the study, with a minimum of four years follow-up. (Delamarter et al, 2010) Demographic data remained similar between the arthroplasty and ACDF groups. All clinical parameters improved equally in both groups at all follow-up periods (p<.0001). A significant difference in the study was the rate of secondary surgical procedures. At the four year follow-up point, 12 (11.3%) of the ACDF patients had additional surgery, while only three (2.9%) of the ProDisc-C patients required further procedures (p=.0292). The ACDF patients primarily required additional surgery for pseudoarthrosis at the index level; however, six (5.6%) ACDF patients had surgery at an adjacent level. Three ProDisc-C patients were converted to fusion for axial pain. No ProDisc-C patients had to have surgery at adjacent levels. In the continued access arm of the study, one ProDisc-C patient required additional surgery to reposition the implant and two were converted to fusion for axial neck pain.

Pimenta et al (Pimenta et al, 2007) prospectively evaluated patients undergoing the PCM cervical disc replacement. Seventy-one single-level and 69 multi-level arthroplasties were performed. While both groups improved, the multi-level patients showed improved scores compared to the single-level patients. The mean NDI improvement was better in the multi-level PCM group (p=0.021). While the overall IDE results have yet to be reported, Philips et al (Phillips et al, 2009) showed in a small set of the IDE patients that arthroplasty was viable at levels adjacent to a prior fusion.

5. Radiographic results

Heterotopic ossification (HO) has initially been reported in the Bryan Cervical Disc Replacement (Bartels & Donk, 2005; Leung et al 2005; Solas et al, 2005) but as the literature expands, no disc arthroplasty has proven immune to this problem. (Figure 7) McAfee et al characterized the severity of HO with a simple scale, modified from lumbar disc arthroplasty findings. The scale ranged from grade 0 (no HO) to grade IV -(complete ankylosis). (McAfee et al, 2003) (Table 2) Delamarter et al described three patients that developed grade IV HO in the ProDisc-C IDE study by 24 months, with two additional patients developing grade IV HO by 48 months. Non-steroidal anti-inflammatory drugs (NSAIDs) were not part of the study protocol. Interestingly in the continued access arm of the study, in which NSAIDs were more commonly used, no patients developed ankylosis at the index level (Delamarter et al, 2010) Mehren et al (Mehren et al, 2006) evaluated the rate of HO at two centers performing cervical disc arthroplasty. Approximately one third of patients postoperatively showed no sign of HO, while almost 20% of patients had HO that lead to restrictions in motion. Nine percent of the patients had grade IV HO, with most of the patients having had multilevel procedures. There was a difference in the overall rate of grade IV HO between the two centers, 12.8% versus 5.2%. The center with the lower HO

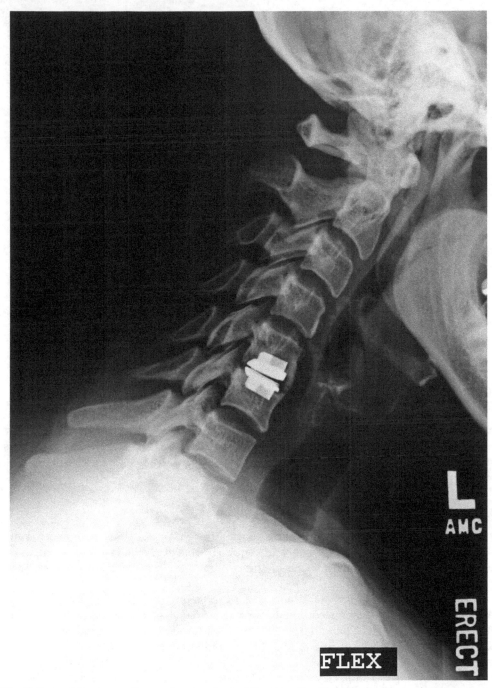

Fig. 7. Lateral flexion radiography- implanted ProDisc-C with heterotopic ossification, preserved motion.

rate routinely prescribed NSAID use postoperatively. Yi et al (Yi et al, 2010) studied the rate of HO according to the arthroplasty type. They found the following HO rates: Bryan 21.0%, Mobi-C (LDR Medical, Troyes, France) 52.5% and ProDisc-C 71.4%. The only two patients that developed grade IV HO were in the Bryan group. All patients routinely received postoperative NSAIDs.

Grade 0	No HO present
Grade I	HO is detectable in front of the vertebral body but not in the anatomic interdiscal space
Grade II	HO is growing in to the disc space. Possible affection of the function of the prosthesis
Grade III	Bridging ossifications which still allow movement of the prosthesis
Grade IV	Complete fusion of the treated segment without movement in flexion/extension

HO indicates Heterotopic ossification

(modified from McAfee et al, 2003)

Table 2. Characterisation of the Different Grades of Heterotopic Ossification (HO) in Total Cervical Disc Replacement

In all the clinical studies evaluating cervical disc arthroplasty and HO, there has been no correlation between the development of HO and the clinical results. Barbargallo et al (Barbargallo et al, 2010) specifically looked at this aspect of cervical disc arthroplasty. They found an overall rate of HO development of 42% and no difference in the functional scores in patients with or without HO. Segmental range of motion of $\geq 3°$ was preserved in 93.8% of patients with HO.

6. Complications

All of the large clinical series published on cervical disc arthroplasty have not reported any severe neurological injuries, such as quadriplegia. The rate of revision surgery at the index level has been acceptably low. None of the cervical disc arthroplasty series have had implants removed for infection.

Concerns of wear debris and local and remote inflammatory changes in cervical disc arthroplasty have been expressed. *In vitro* wear tests have been submitted to the United States FDA as part of the clinical approval process. Generally, wear debris volume has been in the range of 10% of that produced by large joint arthroplasties. Anderson et al (Anderson et al 2004) published *in vitro* wear testing on the Bryan Cervical Disc Replacement using a custom cervical spine simulator on six disc assemblies. At 10 million cycles, the mean mass loss was 1.76% and a mean height loss of 0.75%. At 40 million cycles there was an 18% mass loss. Wear particles were elliptical in shape and larger than typical particles in large joint arthroplasties. Anderson studied local and remote wear debris and the subsequent inflammatory response using an *in vivo* caprine model with implanted Bryan arthroplasties. Sacrificed animals at up to twelve months showed an increase in extracellular wear debris. No apparent inflammatory response was seen locally or distally in these animals.

Clinically, there have been scattered case reports of osteolysis after cervical disc arthroplasty implantation. Tumialan and Gluf reported on a 30-year-old man who underwent a ProDisc-C arthroplasty at C5-6. (Tumialan & Gluf, 2011) He had an uneventful postoperative course until he developed worsening neck pain at nine months. Repeat imaging studies by 15 months showed a progressive osteolysis process in the vicinity of the superior endplate and keel. Work-up for infection was negative. The patient underwent explantation of the arthroplasty and conversion to a fusion. The implant was studied after removal and no defects or unusual wear was noted. The authors hypothesized that the most likely cause of the osteolysis was an immune mediated process. Longer study periods are needed to determine the significance of wear changes and the rate of osteolysis of cervical disc arthroplasty.

7. Conclusions

Cervical disc arthroplasty has been one of the most closely scrutinized surgical procedures in the last decade. Short-term prospective clinical studies show cervical disc arthroplasty to be at least the equivalent of ACDF for degenerative pathology. There is some evidence that cervical disc arthroplasty may play a role in diminishing adjacent segment disease. However, the long-term efficacy and safety of cervical disc arthroplasty await further clinical studies.

8. References

[1] Amevo B, Worth D, Bogduk N. (1991) Instantaneous axis of rotation of the typical cervical motion segments: a study in normal volunteers. *Clinical Biomechanics* Vol. 6: pp. 111-117

[2] Anderson PA, Sasso RC, Rouleau JP et al. (2004) The Bryan Cervical Disc: wear properties and early clinical results. *Spine Journal*, 4(6): 5303-5309

[3] Bailey R, Badgely C. (1960) Stabilization of the cervical spine by anterior fusion. *Journal of Bone and Joint Surgery Am*, 42(4): 565-594

[4] Barbargallo GM, Corbino LA, Olindo G, et al. (2010) Heterotopic ossification in cervical disc arthroplasty: Is it clinically relevant? *Evidence-Based Spine Care Journal*, 1(1):15-20

[5] Bartels RH, Donk R. (2005) Fusion around cervical disc prosthesis: Case report. *Neurosurgery*, 57:E194

[6] Bogduk N, Mercer S. (2000) *Clinical Biomechanics*, 15(9): 633-648

[7] Bohlman HH, Emery SE, Goodfellow DB, et al. (1993) Robinson anterior cervical discectomy and arthrodesis for cervical radiculopathy: long term follow-up of one hundred and twenty-two patients. *Journal of Bone and Joint Surgery Am*, 75: 1298-1307

[8] Cloward RD. (1961) Treatment of acute fractures and fracture dislocations of cervical spine by vertebral body fusion: a report of cases. *Journal of Neurosurgery*, 118: 205-209

[9] Cummins BH, Robertson JT, Gill SS. (1998) Surgical experience with an implanted artificial cervical joint. *Journal of Neurosurgery*, 88: 943-948

[10] Delamarter RB, Pradhan BB. (2004) Indications for cervical spine prostheses, early experiences with ProDisc-C in the USA. *Spine Art*, 1:7-9

[11] Delamarter RB, Murrey D, Janssen MI et al. (2010) Results of 24 months from the prospective, randomized, multicenter investigation device exemption trial of ProDisc-C versus anterior cervical discectomy and fusion with 4-year follow-up and continued access patients. *SAS Journal*, 4: 122-128

[12] DiAngelo DJ, Robertson JT, Metcalf NH et al. (2003) Biomechanical testing of an artificial cervical joint and an anterior cervical plate. *Journal of Spinal Disorders and Tech*, 16(4): 314-323

[13] Dmitriev AE, Cunningham BW, Hu N et al. (2005) Adjacent level intradiscal pressure and segmental kinematics following a cervical total disc arthroplasty: An in vitro human cadaveric model. *Spine*, 30: 1165-1172

[14] Dvorak J, Panjabi MM, Grob D et al. (1993) Clinical validation of functional flexion/extension radiographs of the cervical spine. *Spine*, 18:120-127

[15] Dvorak J, Panjabi MM, Novotny JE et al. (1991) In vivo flexion/extension of the normal cervical spine. *Journal of Orthop Res*, 9: 828-834

[16] Eck JC, Humphreys SC, Lim T, et al. (2002) Biomechanical study on the effect of cervical spine fusion on adjacent level intradiscal pressure and segment motion. *Spine*, 27: 2431-2434

[17] Goffin J, VanLoo J, VanCalenbergh F et al. (2010) A clinical analysis of 4-6 year follow-up results after cervical disc replacement using the Bryan Cervical Disc Prosthesis. *J Neurosurgery Spine*, 12 (3) 261-9

[18] Goffin J, Geusens E, Vantomme N, et al. (2004) Long-term follow-up after interbody fusion of the cervical spine. *Journal of Spinal Disorders and Techniques*, 17(2) 79-85

[19] Goffin J, Casey A, Kehr P, et al. (2002) Preliminary clinical experience with the Bryan cervical disc prosthesis. *Neurosurgery*, 51(3) 840-845.

[20] Goffin J, Van Loon J, VanCalenbergh F, et al. (1995) Long-term results after anterior cervical fusion and osteosynthetic stabilization for fractures and/or dislocation of the cervical spine. *Journal of Spinal Disorders and Techniques*, 8: 500-508

[21] Gore DR, Sepic SB. (1998) Anterior discectomy and fusion for painful cervical disc disease: a report of 50 patients with an average follow-up of 21 years. *Spine*, 23: 2047-2051

[22] Gore DR, Sepic SB. (1984) Anterior cervical fusion for degenerated or protruded discs: A review of one hundred forty-six patients. *Spine*, 9:667-71

[23] Heller JG, Sasso RC, Papadopoulos SM, Anderson PA, Fessler RG et al. (2009) Comparison of Bryan Cervical Disc Arthroplasty with anterior cervical decompression and fusion. *Spine*, 34(2) 101- 107

[24] Huang RC, Girardi FP, Cammisa FP et al. (2003) The implications of constraint in lumbar total disc replacement. *Journal of Spinal Disorders and Techniques*, 16(4): 412-417

[25] Hilibrand AS, Carlson GD, Palumbo MA, et al. (1999) Radiculopathy and myelopathy at segments adjacent to the site of a previous anterior cervical arthrodesis. *Journal of Bone and Joint Surgery Am*, 81: 519-528

[26] Mehren, Suchomel et al. (2006) Heterotopic ossification in total cervical artificial disc replacement. *Spine*, 31(24) 2802-2806

[27] Leung C, Casey et al. (2005) Clinical significance of Heterotopic ossification in cervical disc replacement: a prospective multi-center clinical trial. *Neurosurgery*, 57:759-631 discussion 763

[28] McAfee, Cunningham et al. (2003) Classification of Heterotopic ossification (HO) in artificial disk replacement. *Journal of Spinal Disorders and Techniques* 16: 384-9

[29] Mummaneni et al. Clinical and radiographic analysis of cervical disc arthroplasty compared with allograft fusion: A randomized controlled trial. *Journal of Neurosurgery –Spine*, Vol. 6, pp 198-209

[30] Murrey et al. (2009) Results of the prospective, randomized, controlled Food and Drug Administration Investigational Device Exemption Study of the ProDisc-C total disc replacement versus anterior discectomy and fusion for the treatment of one level symptomatic cervical disc disease. *Spine Journal*, Vol. 9, pp 275-286

[31] Peng CW, Yue WM, Abdul B et al. (2011) Intermediate results of the Prestige LP cervical disc replacement: clinical and radiological analysis with minimum two-year follow-up. *Spine*, 36 (2): E 105-111

[32] Pospiech J, Stolke D, Wilke HJ et al. (1999) Intradiscal pressure recordings in the cervical spine. *Neurosurgery*, 44: 379-384.

[33] Phillips FM, Allen TR, Regen JJ, et al. (2009) Cervical disc replacement in patients with and without previous adjacent level fusion surgery: A prospective study. *Spine*, 34 (6) 556-565

[34] Pimenta L, McAfee PC, Cappuccino A, et al. (2007) Superiority of multilevel cervical arthroplasty outcomes versus single level outcomes: 229 consecutive PCM prostheses. *Spine*, 32 (12) 1337-1344

[35] Penning L. (1978) Normal movements of the cervical spine. *Am J Roentgenol*, 130: 317-326

[36] Raposo J, Darden BV. (publication pending) Biomechanics of cervical disc arthroplasty. *The Cervical Spine, 5th Edition*. Editor Edward Benzel, Lippincott, Williams and Wilkins

[37] Riew KD, Buchowski JM, Sasso R, Zdeblick T, Metcalf NH, Anderson PA. (2008) Cervical disc arthroplasty compared with arthrodesis for the treatment of myelopathy. *Journal of Bone and Joint-A*, Vol. 90: pp 2354-2364

[38] Robinson R, Smith G. (1955): Anterolateral cervical disc removal and interbody fusion for cervical disc syndrome. *Bull. John Hopkins Hospital*, 96:223-224

[39] Sola S, Hebecker R, Knoop M et al. (2005 suppl) Bryan cervical disc prosthesis- three years follow-up. *European Spine Journal*, 14:38

[40] Tumialan LM and Gluf, Wm. (2011) Progressive vertebral body osteolysis after cervical arthroplasty. *Spine*, 36(14):973-8

[41] Yi S, Kim KN, Yang MS, et al. (2010)   Difference in occurrence of Heterotopic ossification according to prosthesis type in the cervical artificial disc replacement. *Spine*, 35(16):1556-1561

7

Shoulder Hemiarthroplasty in Proximal Humerus Fractures

José Hernández Enríquez, Xavier A. Duralde and Antonio J. Pérez Caballer
¹Orthopaedics Department, Hospital Infanta Elena, Valdemoro
²Orthopaedics Department, Peachtree Orthopaedic Clinic, Atlanta GA
³Orthopaedics Department, Hospital Infanta Elena, Valdemoro
¹,³Spain
²USA

1. Introduction

We present a review of the most recent published articles related to shoulder hemiarthroplasty in proximal humerus fractures. Four-part proximal humerus fractures represent between 2% and 10% of all proximal fractures where displacement occurs as a result of the muscular deforming force.

Hemiarthroplasty is indicated in patients with four-part fractures and in elderly patients with osteoporotic bone who have fracture-dislocations. In both groups of patients, obtaining a secure stable reduction using internal fixation techniques is difficult, and the rate of osteonecrosis can range from 13% to 35% in four-part fractures. Hemiarthroplasty can also be considered in patients with three-part fractures and fracture-dislocations when bone quality is poor and the degree of conminution precludes satisfactory reduction and internal fixation. Headsplitting proximal humerus fractures in elderly patients also should be treated with hemiarhroplasty. Primary replacement can be considered in younger patients with four-part proximal fractures if acceptable redution cannot be obtained.

The important surgical principles when performing a hemiartroplasty for four-part proximal humeral fractures include the following: the use of a deltopectoral approach, allowing preservation of the deltoid origin and insertion; restoration of humeral length and retroversion; and secure fixation of the tuberosities to the prosthesis, to the shaft and to one another.

Results of hemiarthroplasty for four-part proximal humerus fractures are somewhat difficult to interpret, specifically because other proximal humerus fracture patterns often are included in published series. Wide variation in outcomes measurements also makes comparisons between studies difficult. Despite these limitations, hemiarthroplasty offers reliable pain relief and reasonable levels of patient satisfaction, but only modest functional results. Limited use with activities of daily living below shoulder level may be reliably obtained but overhead use is not typical following this surgery.

Significant residual pain generally tends to be associated with moderate activity: minimal pain occurs at rest. Even when motion and functional results are limited, pain relief is reported to be consistent.

Reports of patient satisfaction vary widely, in part because of the numerous scales used to measure outcomes and satisfaction. High satisfaction rates seem to correlate more with pain relief than with range of motion of functional outcomes. Even studies with poor functional results report high patient satisfaction if pain relief is acceptable.

The prognostic factors have been shown to be the age, the delay between injury and surgery, preoperative neurologic deficit, history of cigarette smoking, excessive alcohol consumption and female sex. Tuberosity position and healing may be the most important factors in determining outcome.

Recently the use of the Reverse Total Shoulder Replacement has been recommended in selected cases of proximal humeral fracture. Although the indications and results of this technique are not well known yet, this may offer an advantage in selected cases over traditional Humeral Head Replacement. Any possible advantages of this technique must be weighed against increased risks and the known results of humeral head replacement.

Humeral head replacement is indicated for a select group of proximal humeral fractures depending on the severity and pattern of the fracture as well as bone quality and cuff integrity (Compito et al 1994). The results of this surgery are dependent on patient factors, timing of surgery, and technical factors associated with the performance of the operation. The majority of fractures of the proximal humerus can be treated nonoperatively but a full 15% of cases will require some type of operative interventio (Young et al 1985, Zuckerman et al 2007). Neer's fracture classification has generally served as a reliable guide to fracture managemen (Neer et al 1970, 1970). The more severe the injury, the higher the risk of avascular necrosis of the humeral head, malunion, or nonunion of the fracture. When indicated, early surgical intervention leads to superior results and avoids many complications associated with delayed management (Demirhan et al 2003, Duralde & Leddy 2010).

Operative treatment options for proximal humeral fractures include various forms of open or closed reduction and fixation versus prosthetic replacement. The introduction of the proximal humeral locking plate has expanded the indications for ORIF as patients with osteoporotic bone can now be better managed utilizing this plate for fixation (Duralde & Leedy 2010). Even cases of late avascular necrosis following ORIF can be managed effectively with hardware removal and prosthetic replacement as long as the tuberosities have healed in a relatively anatomic position (Boileau et al 2001). Similarly advances in the technique of closed reduction and percutaneous pinning have increased the indications for this modality (Jaberg et al 1992). ORIF remains a good option for displaced 2-part fractures, 3-part fractures (even in the face of osteoporosis), and impacted valgus 4-part fractures of the proximal humerus (Bastian & Hertel 2009, Duralde & Leedy 2010). Four-part fractures in young patients are preferably treated with a locking plate but if stable fixation cannot be attained, humeral head replacement is indicated. A group of fractures remain, however, that are not amenable to this modality and require prosthetic replacement for adequate management.

Prosthetic replacement for proximal humeral fractures remains the treatment of choice for 4-part fracture dislocations, head-split fractures, and head impaction fractures of >40%. These fractures represent between 2 and 10% of proximal humeral fractures (Zuckerman & Sajadi 2007). It remains a good option in comminuted 3-part fractures especially in elderly patients with poor bone quality or a high degree of comminution (Bigliani 1990). Humeral head replacement is contraindicated in cases of active infection, severe nerve palsy to the deltoid and rotator cuff, and in patients unable to comply with the postoperative rehabilitation program. In patients with known chronic large rotator cuff tears, the results of humeral head replacement for fracture are poor (Compito et al 1994) and this may be an indication for the use of a Reverse Total Shoulder Arthroplasty (RTSA). Indications and technical recommendations for the use of the RTSA in this setting are not clearly defined but this represents an area of exciting new research (Franke et al 2002, Wall & Walch 2007).

Prosthetic replacement for proximal humerus fractures is a challenging operation with variable results reported in the orthopaedic literature especially in terms of patient function (Robinson et al 2003). This procedure is performed uncommonly even by shoulder specialists. Anatomic landmarks are lost due to fracture of the tuberosities away from the humeral shaft making proper placement of prosthesis in terms of height and version a challenge. Tuberosities may be comminuted and the deforming pull of the rotator cuff tendons represents a challenge to fracture healing. Excellent results following humeral head replacement for fracture are associated with proper implant selection and insertion, anatomic tuberosity healing, and early rehabilitation to restore motion and strength[3]. Conversely, poor results are most commonly associated with tuberosity malunion or nonunion and improper humeral stem positioning (Bolileau et al 2002, Demirhan et al 2003, Esen et al 2009, Frankle et al 2001, Robinson et al 2003). Other important factors include the timing of surgery, patient age, tobacco and alcohol use, and female sex. Despite intensive study and improvements in patient selection, prosthetic design, and surgical technique, functional results remain variable. Wide variation in outcomes measurements also makes comparisons between studies difficult. Despite these limitations, hemiarthroplasty offers reliable pain relief and reasonable levels of patient satisfaction, but only modest functional results. Limited use with activities of daily living below shoulder level may be reliably obtained but overhead use is not typical following this surgery. Good to excellent results remain between 75-85% despite these challenges (Bigliani 1990, Goldman et al 1995, Green et al 1993, Kontakis et al 2008, Moeckel et al 1992, Robinson et al 2003, Tanner & Cofield 1983). High satisfaction rates seem to correlate more with pain relief than with range of motion or functional outcomes. Even studies with poor functional results report high patient satisfaction if pain relief is acceptable. Certainly, the more prepared the surgeon finds him or herself in the management of the patient with a severely displaced proximal humeral fracture, the better the chance of success. The purpose of this article is to review the preoperative evaluation, describe the surgical technique required for successful placement of the prosthesis and fixation of the tuberosities, and outline a safe postoperative rehabilitation program. We will review current results and complications associated with the technique of humeral head replacement and Reverse total shoulder arthroplasty for proximal humeral fractures.

2. Shoulder arthroplasty for proximal humerus fractures

2.1 Preoperative evaluation

Adequate preoperative evaluation is critical in the management of patients with displaced proximal humerus fractures. The surgeon must have a good working knowledge as to the mechanism of injury and level of energy associated as this will give an indication of possible neurovascular injuries. The surgeon should attempt to determine whether the injury represents a fracture or a fracture/dislocation and evaluation of all available radiographic studies is beneficial. Previous history of osteoporosis will give an indication as to the quality of bone available for fixation. Past history of rotator cuff disease is helpful as a large rotator cuff tear will be associated with poor results with a humeral head replacement and may be an indication for reverse ball and socket prosthesis.

Physical examination may be limited in the acute fracture setting because of pain and swelling. The area of bruising is most commonly seen in the chest as well as the arm distal to the deltoid muscle. Bruising in the area of the deltoid itself is indicative of either direct trauma to this area or perforation of the deltoid by one of the fracture fragments. Neurovascular examination is typically limited because of pain and the status of the axillary nerve often cannot be determined prior to surgery. Distal pulses should be evaluated and compared to the contralateral side. Differences in distal pulses may be an indication for arteriogram. Displacement of the shaft medially in the area of the brachial plexus is also in indication to obtain an arteriogram prior to open reduction internal fixation. Range of motion testing is of no benefit in the acute fracture setting.

Radiographic examination should be limited to a trauma series which does not require the patient to move the arm. Three orthogonal views as described by Neer can adequately evaluate the fracture in the majority of cases (Neer 1990). (Figure 1) These include an AP view in the scapular plane, a transthoracic lateral view, and a Valpeau axillary view. All of these X-rays can be taken without removal of the arm from the sling. CT scan has been shown to improve the accuracy of fracture classification and is very beneficial in preoperative planning (Shrader et al 2005). (Figure 2)

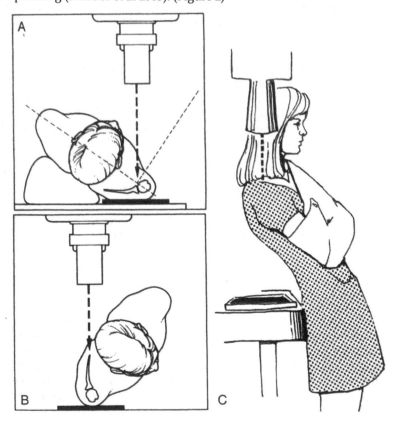

Fig. 1.

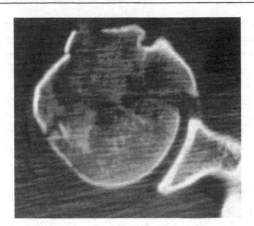

Fig. 2.

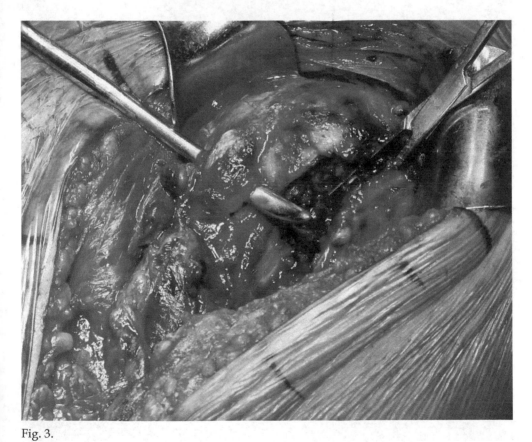

Fig. 3.

Arthroplasty for proximal humerus fractures is typically indicated for head split and head indentation fractures ›40% fractures, displaced 4-part fractures of the proximal humerus, and 4-part fracture/dislocations. In these cases, the proximal humerus does fracture in a very characteristic pattern. The fracture line between the greater and lesser tuberosity typically lies directly posterior to the bicipital groove so that the lesser tuberosity fracture typically also contains the bicipital groove and a small portion of the greater tuberosity. (Figure 3) The remainder of the greater tuberosity often fractures away from the shaft and lesser tuberosity with a characteristic "V" shaped pattern of bone leaving a distinctive defect in the proximal shaft which can be used in realigning the fracture fragments anatomically. (Figure 4) Variable amounts of head fragment may still be attached to a tuberosities. A small portion of the calcar typically stays attached to the humeral head fragment. (Figure 5)

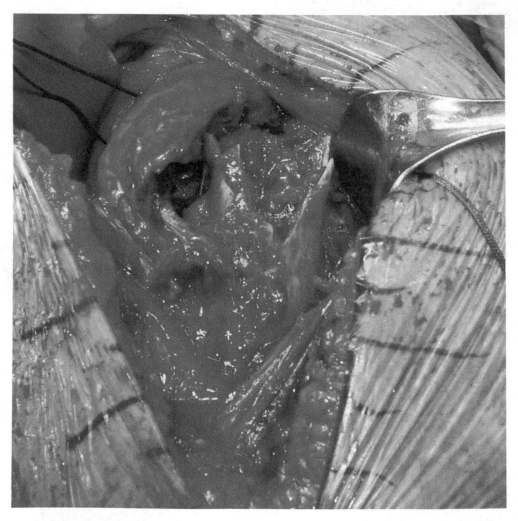

Fig. 4.

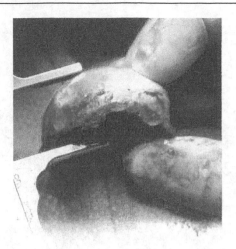

Fig. 5.

2.2 Operative technique

Key goals in prosthetic replacement for proximal humerus fractures include atraumatic exposure of the fracture site with protection of the deltoid origin and insertion while avoiding further devascularization of the fracture fragments, proper positioning of the prosthesis both in terms of height and version, and secure anatomic fixation of the tuberosities. The exact indications for the use of reverse prosthesis in the management of proximal humerus fractures is not well understood currently and is undergoing a period of development and research. Surgery is recommended within 7-10 days after the patient is cleared medically. Delay beyond this time makes dissection more challenging due to early fibrosis. Surgery must be followed by a safe physical therapy program which allows adequate healing of the tuberosities while avoiding excessive stiffness.

This surgery is typically performed under interscalene block anesthesia and general anesthesia. Relaxation during surgery decreases the pull of the pectoralis major and improves exposure. Interscalene block is contraindicated in the face of documented neurologic injury. This block results in excellent postoperative pain relief when indicated. The patient is placed in the beach chair position with the back of the table elevated approximately 30°. The patient is placed at the edge of the operating table with a bolster along the medial border of the scapula to stabilize this structure during surgery. Lateral placement of the arm allows extension off of the table for exposure and access to the humeral shaft. A well-padded neurosurgical head rest allows increased exposure and access to the superior shoulder and a short arm board supports the elbow without blocking access to the arm. All bony prominences are well-padded. A fluoroscan is utilized from above to allow evaluation of the fracture itself and tuberosity positioning. (Figure 6) Broad-spectrum antibiotics are routinely used. Surgical approach is planned to contribute minimal additional trauma to the soft tissues and vascular structures in the area of the proximal humerus. In situations in which the humeral head is displaced into the axilla in the area of the brachial plexus, caution must be exercised in its removal as this can result in hemorrhage. Assistance from a vascular surgeon may be required in such cases.

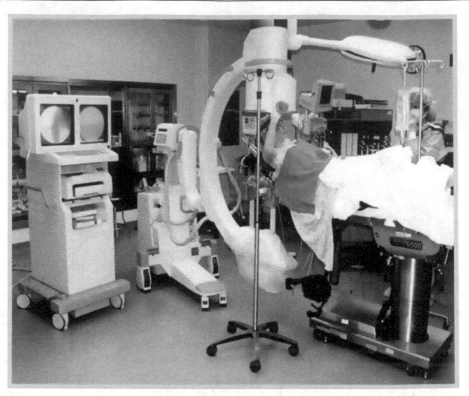

Fig. 6.

2.3 Surgical exposure

A deltopectoral incision is made beginning at the level superior to the coracoid and passing to a point directly anterior to the deltoid insertion. (Figure 7) The fat stripe over the cephalic vein is identified and carefully incised avoiding injury to the vein. With the edema encountered in acute fractures, blunt dissection can be carried through the deltopectoral interval dissecting the cephalic vein laterally with the deltoid down to the level of the fracture site itself. Fracture hematoma is evacuated and the anatomy of the fracture is now examined. The conjoined tendon is retracted medially and the deltoid is retracted laterally. The deltoid origin and insertion are preserved. Landmarks which assist in identification of critical structures include the coracoid which has been named "the lighthouse of the glenoid" and the biceps tendon which has been called "the highway to the glenoid". The coracoacromial ligament is identified at the lateral edge of the coracoid and can be followed to the subacromial space. The base of the coracoid can be palpated and helps guide the surgeon to the glenoid. The biceps tendon can be identified in the pectoralis insertion on the humeral shaft and followed into the fracture site. The fracture line between the lesser and greater tuberosities is typically immediately posterior to this tendon. The axillary nerve must be identified and protected throughout the procedure. The nerve is palpated anteriorly along the inferior border of the subscapularis and laterally along the undersurface of the deltoid muscle. Continuity of this nerve can be verified using the Tug Test (Flatow & Bigliani 1992) and is reassuring that the nerve has not been lacerated by fracture fragments.

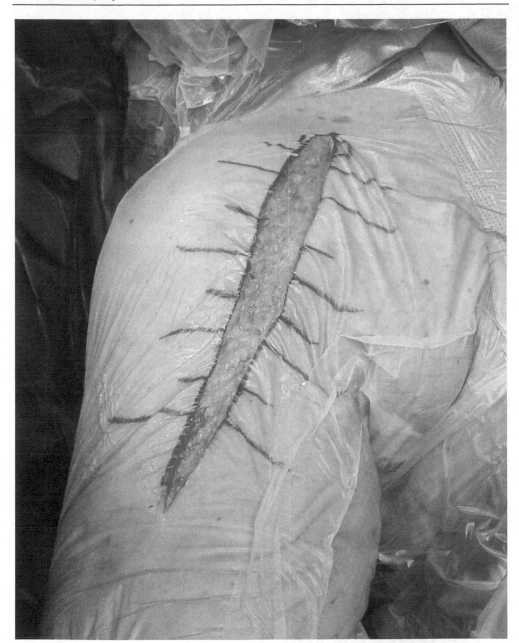

Fig. 7.

2.4 Control of fracture

The first step in controlling the 4-part proximal humerus fracture is to control the tuberosities. The lesser tuberosity is displaced medially by the pull of the subscapularis while the greater tuberosity is displaced posterosuperiorly by the pull of the infraspinatus and teres minor muscles. Heavy nonabsorbable sutures are passed through the subscapularis tendon to control the lesser tuberosity and through the infraspinatus tendon to control the greater tuberosity. (Figure 8) A bone hook or clamp may be necessary to reduce the greater tuberosity so that a suture can be passed through the cuff tendon. Abduction of the humerus relaxes the deltoid and assists with exposure of the greater tuberosity. Sutures are not placed through the greater tubersoity itself as bone quality may be poor and this will lead to further comminution. The rotator cuff tendon is often stronger than the bone itself and should be utilized for both mobilization and later fixation. The fracture line between the tuberosities is followed up to the rotator cuff. The rotator cuff can then be split in line with its fibers in continuity with this fracture line. This will leave a small strip of supraspinatus tendon attached to the anterior fragment. This fragment includes the lesser tuberosity, bicipital groove, and a small portion of the greater tuberosity. Attached to it are the subscapularis tendon, the rotator interval, and a small strip of the

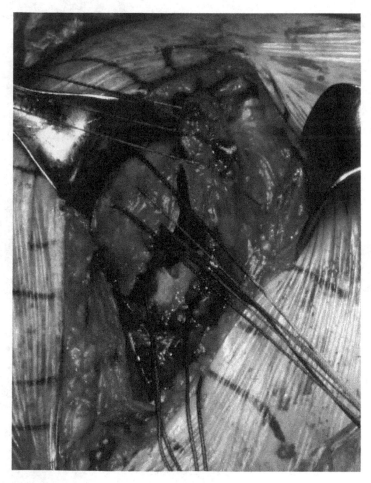

Fig. 8.

supraspinatus tendon. The remainder of the supraspinatus as well as the entire infraspinatus and teres minor tendons will be attached to the posterior fragment. Splitting the supraspinatus in line with its fibers to the level of the glenoid now allows exposure of the glenoid as well as the humeral head.

The humeral head is now removed and placed on the back table where it can be measured in terms of height and diameter. (Figure 9) Any missing fragments from the humeral head are typically still connected to the tuberosities and must be removed to allow adequate reduction of these tuberosities under the prosthetic humeral head. Removal of these portions of the humeral head is necessary but debulking of the tuberosity fragments is contraindicated as this may compromise tuberosity healing and positioning. The humeral head is also carefully inspected to determine the amount of calcar attached medially. The size of this fragment is indicative of the amount of missing shaft medially and will help determine the exact positioning of the prosthesis. The prosthetic humeral head should be positioned superior to the shaft a distance equal to the amount of the calcar bone left attached to the humeral head. Placement of the humeral head directly onto the humeral shaft ignoring the size of this calcar fragment will result in positioning of the head too low relative to the shaft. All cancellous bone in the humeral head can now be harvested and used for bone grafting of the tuberosities prior to fixation.

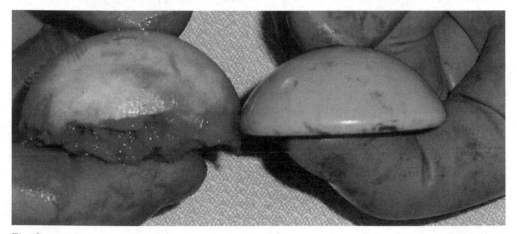

Fig. 9.

2.5 Prosthetic selection

Adequate prosthetic selection is determined by measuring the humeral head and canal. The proximal humeral shaft can be delivered into the operative site by extension, adduction and external rotation of the arm and placement of the elbow onto the short arm board. This allows access to the proximal humeral canal which can be measured with reamers. Minimal reaming is required. If there is no significant shaft comminution associated with the fracture, a standard length prosthetic stem on the order of 130 mm is adequate and a long stem prosthesis is not required. A prosthetic system which allows use of a narrow stem is preferred as this will allow room for bone grafting and tuberosity reduction and healing. Prostheses with a broad proximal collar often do not allow enough room for tuberosity reduction without debulking and compromises the healing ability of these tuberosities. Ingrowth material on the proximal stem may be beneficial to tuberosity healing. The prosthetic stem must be narrow enough to allow adequate insertion into the humerus and avoid proud placement of the prosthesis. Prosthetic humeral head size is determined by measuring the patient's humeral head at the time of surgery both in terms of height and diameter. In prosthetic systems with an offset humeral head, placement of the maximum offset is recommended posteriorly or posterosuperiorly to allow placement of the greater tuberosity under the humeral head in this location. Appropriate head sizing will help reestablish anatomic tension on the rotator cuff tendons after tuberosity repair.

2.6 Prosthetic positioning

Adequate positioning of the prosthesis both in terms of height and version is critical towards the success of this procedure and in reestablishing relatively normal anatomy for the patient postoperatively. Distortion of the normal proximal humeral anatomy by displacement of the tuberosities represents a challenge for determination of proper stem and head height. This positioning is important to reestablish the normal resting length of the deltoid muscle. There are multiple options for determining adequate height for the prosthesis. The superior margin of the pectoralis insertion typically is 56 mm from the superior aspect of the greater tuberosity and is a fairly standard measurement in patients of varying sizes (Murachovsky et al 2006). This measurement will allow the surgeon to determine whether he is in the generally correct range for prosthetic height. As mentioned previously, the size of the fragment of calcar on the humeral head will indicate the height of the prosthetic head relative to the shaft. In cases in which the greater tuberosity does not have significant comminution, the greater tuberosity fragment can be interdigitated back in the "V" shaped defect just posterior to the bicipital groove. The humeral head must be placed just superior to the greater tuberosity in this location and by reducing the greater tuberosity to the shaft, the surgeon can determine proper head height. (Figure 10[a] and 10[b]) Tension on the biceps tendon has been recommended as a guide for the prosthetic height but is less exact. The biceps can be tenodesed at this time and removed from the joint. Finally, some prosthetic systems do allow preoperative templating relative to the contralateral arm with jigs which can be utilized for determining height. These systems are often unwieldy and difficult to use. Placement of the prosthesis too low will result in inferior subluxation of the humeral head relative to the glenoid and cause weakness in elevation. Proud placement of the prosthesis will lead to overstuffing of the joint, superior subluxation, pain, and stiffness. Anatomic version of the humeral head has been generally reported between 20 and 40° of retroversion. Placing the prosthesis in less retroversion places less tension on the greater tuberosity fragment during internal rotation and may benefit healing. Version of approximately 20° is recommended for this reason and can be determined relative to the patients' forearm. In prosthetic systems with a posterior fin of the prosthesis positioned 180° from the medial calcar portion of the stem, this posterior fin should generally be located just posterior to the bicipital groove. The humeral stem is generally cemented in place to avoid subsidence and malrotation because the stabilizing effect typically afforded by the tuberosities has been lost due to the fracture.

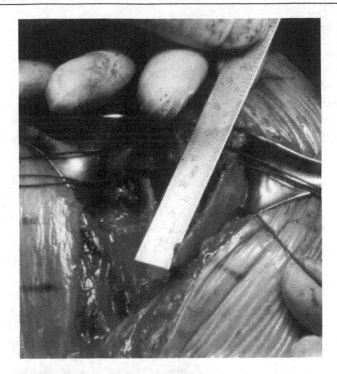

Fig. 10a.

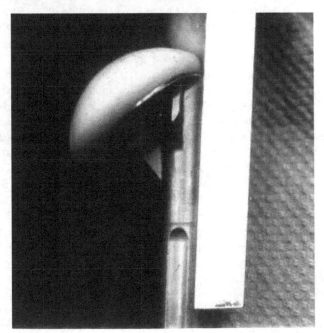

Fig. 10b.

2.7 Tuberosity fixation

Postoperative function is most closely tied to anatomic healing of the tuberosities. The success of tuberosity healing is directly related to the adequacy of reduction and fixation of the tuberosities at the time of surgery. Tuberosity healing is a major challenge and greater tuberosity pull off remains the most common complication of this surgery (Boileau et al 2002). The tuberosities must heal to each other and to the shaft as well as to the ingrowth material of the humeral prosthesis. A variety of fixation techniques have been reported but techniques recommended by both Frankle and Boileau have demonstrated superior biomechanical resistance to deforming forces (Boileau et al 2000, Frankle et al 2002). The tuberosities are repaired utilizing a suture technique which fixes these tuberosities to each other, to the prosthesis, and to the shaft of the humerus. The placement of these sutures and drill holes for their placement is necessary prior to cementing the humeral stem in place. Drill holes in the shaft include the one drill hole anterior to the bicipital groove, two drill holes straddling the bicipital groove, and one drill hole posterior to the bicipital groove. (Figure 11) In cases in which the "V" shaped fragment of the greater tuberosity is of adequate size, small drill holes between this fragment and the humeral shaft just posterior to the bicipital groove can be utilized for a figure of 8 reduction suture. (Figure 12) This suture does not resist deforming forces but is used for anatomic reduction of the tuberosity. #5 polyester nonabsorbable sutures are placed through the anterior drill hole and through the posterior drill hole respectively. One #5 polyester suture is passed through the holes straddling the bicipital groove in such a way that both ends of this suture pass out from the canal with a small loop of suture inside the canal. While the cement for stem fixation is curing, morcelized bone graft is packed into the proximal canal just above the cement. (Figure 13) These small fragments are fixed to the cement while the cement is setting. This creates a bony surface for healing to the tuberosities. The greater tuberosity is repaired first. One or two cerclage sutures of #5 polyester suture are placed through the rotator cuff at the bone tendon junction and around the anterior stem of the prosthesis. The #5 polyester suture from the anterior drill hole in the shaft is then passed diagonally across the prosthesis and through the rotator cuff tendon at the bone-tendon interface to fix the greater tuberosity to the shaft and to resist vertically directed deforming forces against the tuberosity. (Figure 14) The greater tuberosity is fixed to the posterior aspect of the fin on the stem just inferior to the humeral head utilizing the cerclage sutures passed around the prosthesis. The bone graft is inserted between the prosthesis and the greater tuberosity to restore bulk to the tuberosity and to assist with healing. The posterior shaft suture is then passed diagonally across the prosthesis and passed through the subscapularis tendon at the bone-tendon junction. One to two cerclage sutures between the greater tuberosity and lesser tuberosity are then used to reduce the lesser tuberosity to the stem just underneath the humeral head anterior to the prosthetic fin. Again bone graft is used as needed and the cerclage sutures are tied. The suture from the posterior shaft to the lesser tuberosity is then tied. The rotator cuff split made previously during exposure is closed using nonabsorbable figure of 8 sutures. By making that split through the supraspinatus tendon, good tissue is available for repair anteriorly and posteriorly to help resist greater tuberosity pull-off. Finally, the two suture limbs at the bicipital groove distally are passed in a figure of 8 fashion over the rotator interval and rotator cuff split to firmly repair these to each other and to the shaft. (Figure 15) The stability and strength of the repair is then tested by taking the arm through gentle range of motion. (Figure 16) Adequacy of reduction of the tuberosity fragments can be verified fluoroscopically. The continuity of the axillary nerve can be verified using the Tug test. Suction drains are placed deep to the deltoid and a layered closure is performed.

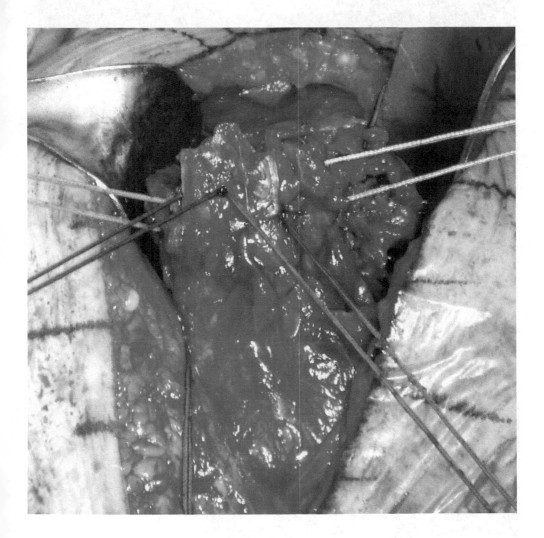

Fig. 11.

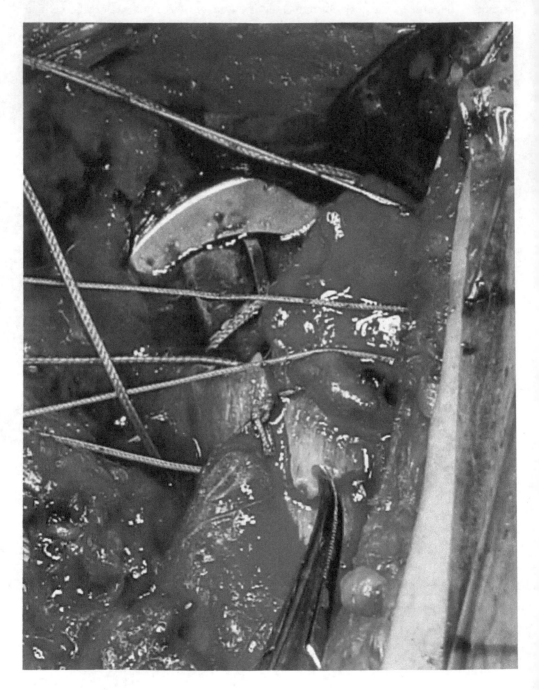

Fig. 12.

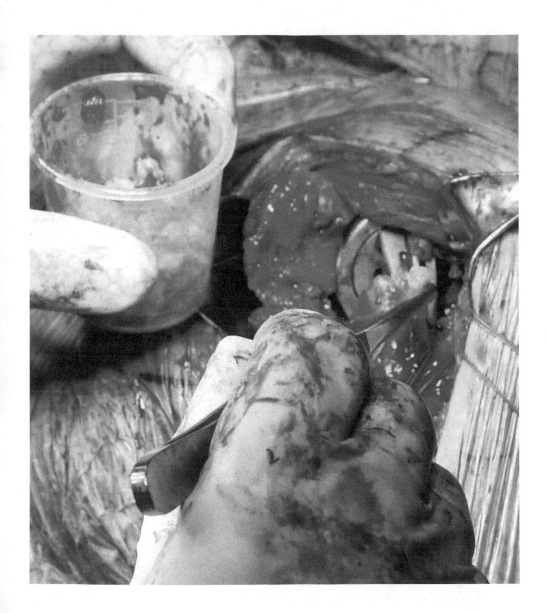

Fig. 13.

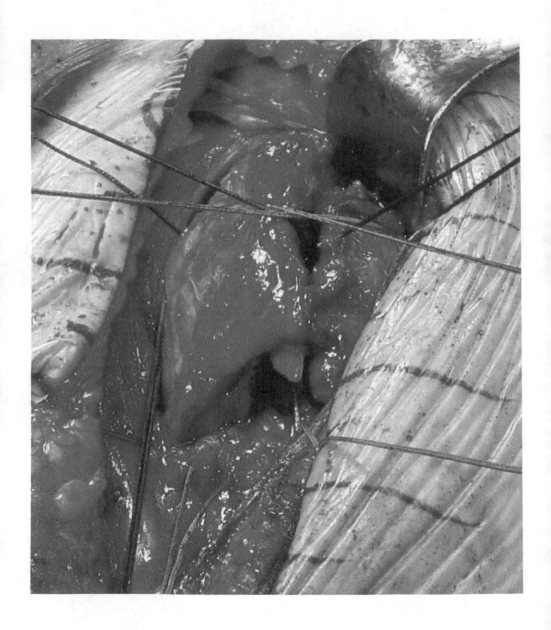

Fig. 14.

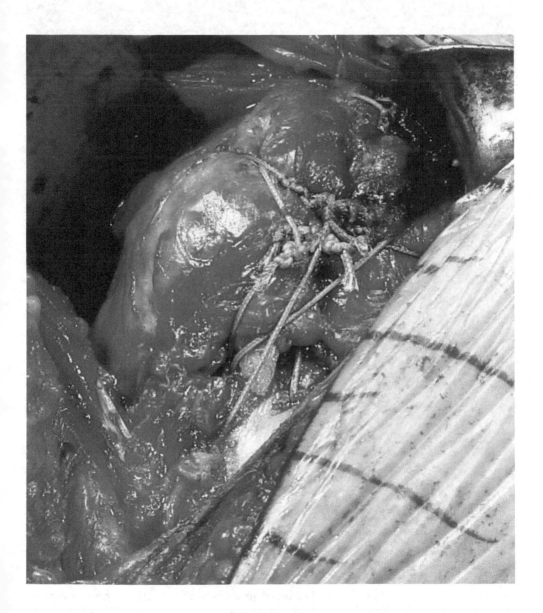

Fig. 15.

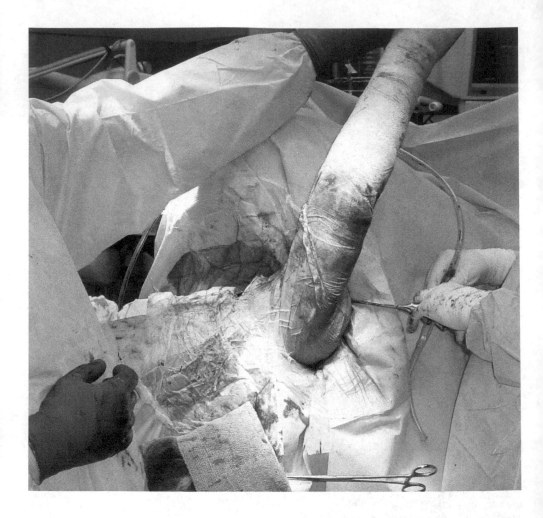

Fig. 16.

2.8 Reverse prosthesis for fracture

Indications for the use of the reverse total shoulder arthroplasty in the management of displaced proximal humerus fractures is in evolution. This prosthesis is generally not recommended in younger patients and it's use has most often been reported in patients around the age of 70. It should be considered in cases with a relatively poor prognosis with use of the humeral head replacement including elderly patients (>75), patients with pre-existing large rotator cuff tears, and patients whose fracture care has been delayed. These patients are at particular risk for poor tuberosity healing (Boileau et al 2002). Use has been spurred by variability in functional results of the humeral head replacement in the management of these complex fractures. The technique of reverse prosthesis in this situation is relatively straightforward (Wall & Walch 2007). The dissection up to removal of the humeral head is identical to that described previously for standard humeral head replacement. The deltopectoral approach is preferred over the superior approach for this indication as it permits easier rehabilitation and allows the surgeon to address any distal humeral shaft comminution that may be present. The exposure of the glenoid is easier than usual as the tuberosities are displaced away from the shaft and the glenoid can be clearly visualized at the time of surgery. The capsule and labrum are released from the glenoid to allow clear exposure of the glenoid rim. The glenoid is reamed according to the specifications of the particular prosthesis. The glenoid baseplate is placed slightly inferiorly and inclined caudally to help avoid notching of the lateral scapular border. Standard placement of the glenosphere is indicated. Humeral stem placement is dictated by soft tissue tension as in standard cases. Minimal or no pistoning of the stem relative to glenosphere should be present with adequate tension across the deltoid. Tension on the tuberosities will also influence the determination of stem height. Version is generally recommended at 0-20° of retroversion but can be altered to allow for optimal tuberosity reduction. In cases in which the supraspinatus is still attached to the greater tuberosity, the tendon insertion may require release in order to mobilize the tuberosity distally enough to reach the shaft and prosthesis. Similar suture fixation is recommended with cerclage sutures between the tuberosities and the prosthesis as well as the vertically aligned sutures diagonally between the shaft and the greater and lesser tuberosities. (Figure 17ª and 17ᵇ) Prostheses with proximal ingrowth may help tuberosity union. Tuberosity repair should decrease incidence of prosthetic instability and allow improved external rotation postoperatively. Currently limited information as to the benefits of tuberosity healing is available in this setting (Bufquin et al 2007). Following tuberosity fixation with either the reverse prosthesis or standard humeral head replacement, suction drainage in indicated to avoid hematoma formation. The deltopectoral interval is closed and the skin is closed in a layered fashion.

Postoperative rehabilitation is geared toward allowing adequate tuberosity healing while helping the patient to regain flexibility in a reasonable and safe fashion. During the first six weeks following surgery the tuberosities are vulnerable to avulsion from active use or extreme range of motion with passive stretching. A protective ultrasling is indicated for the first six weeks following surgery holding the arm in neutral rotation to limit tension on the greater tuberosity fragment. The patient is allowed to perform gentle pendulum exercises with passive external rotation exercises utilizing a stick. Range of motion exercises of the elbow, wrist, and fingers are encouraged with gentle active use of these joints.

Once tuberosity healing can be verified radiographically, active use of the arm can be instituted. This typically occurs at approximately six weeks following surgery. Active-assisted exercises are begun in the supine position along with passive stretching under the supervision of a physical therapist. Light activities of daily living are allowed with the elbow at the side with progression of this as active function increases. Between weeks 6 and 12, exercises are characterized by gentle stretching with isometric strengthening for muscle reeducation. Beginning at 12 weeks, a resistive exercise program can be started below shoulder level with advancement to above shoulder exercises once the patient's strength increases.

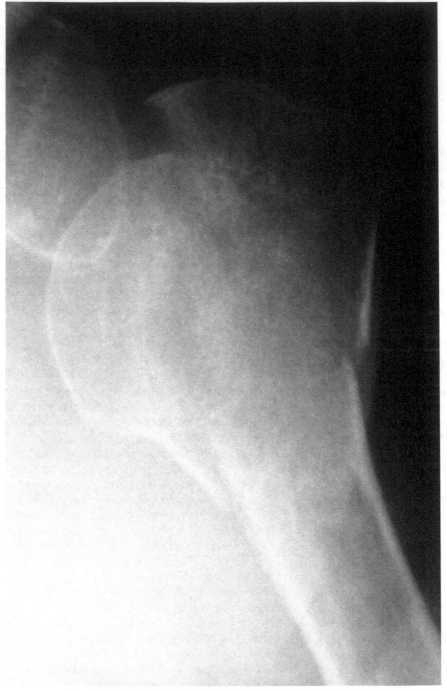

Fig. 17a.

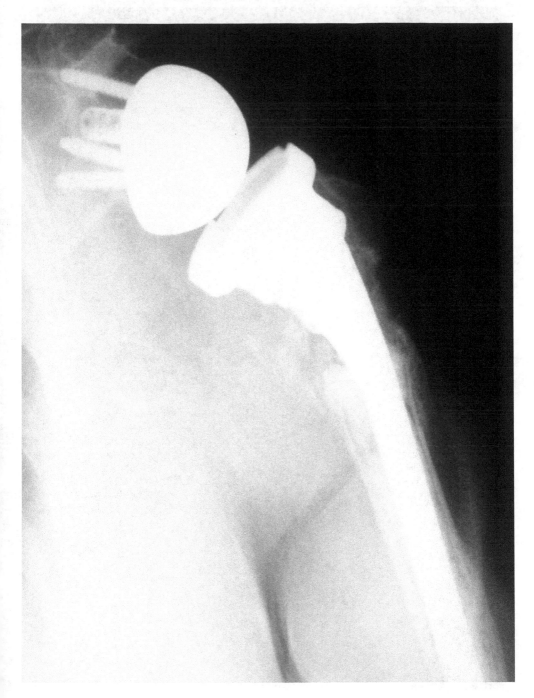

Fig. 17b.

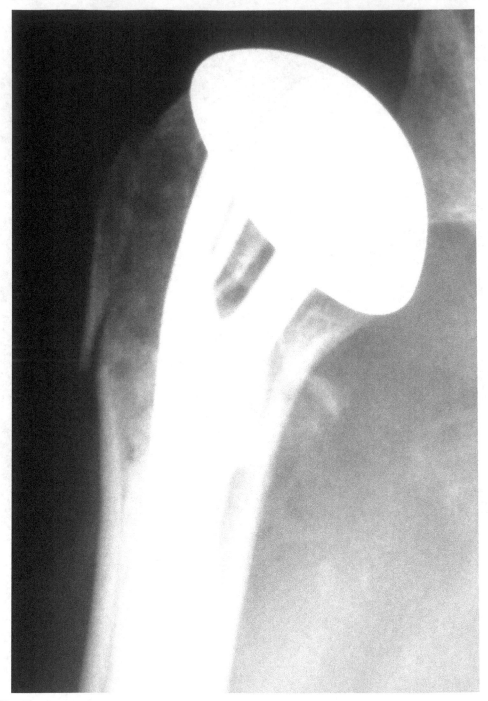

Fig. 18.

3. Results

Complex displaced three and four-part fractures, fracture-dislocations, and fractures with a humeral head split are at risk for the development of malunion and osteonecrosis, especially after internal fixation. Shoulder hemiarthroplasty or, recently, reverse total shoulder arthroplasty is indicated for the treatment of some of these complex fractures (Voos et al 2010).

In spite of advanced patient age, tuberosity healing can be achived by reattachment and bone grafting around specific Reverse Fracture prosthesis, according to Boileau et al. Successful peri-prosthetic tuberosity healing is associated with restoration of both active elevation and external rotation (Boileau et al 2010). (Figure 18)

3.1 Pain relief

Pain relief is the most predictable outcome following hemiarthroplasty for four-part proximal humerus fractures. Many authors have supported this finding, with 61% to 97% of patients reporting complete patiens reporting pain relief. Significant resifual pain generally tends to be associated with moderate activity; minimal pain occurs at rest. Even when motion and functional results are limited, pain relief is reported to be consistent (Young et al 2010).

3.2 Patient satisfaction

Reports of patient satisfaction vary widely, from 58% to 92,% , in part because of the numerous scales used to mesure outcome and satisfaction. High satisfaction rates seem to correlate more with pain relief than with range of motion or functional outcomes. Even studies with poor functional results report high patient satisfaction if pain relief is acceptable (Young et al 2010).

3.3 Prognostic factors

Patient age has been shown to be predictive of outcome. Younger patients have improved results, gaining more rang of motion and a higher level of functional return. These improved results are attributed, in part, to motivation and compliance with postoperative rehabilitation and a more structurally intact rotator cuff.

Another prognostic factor is the delay between injury and surgery. A long delay between the time of injury and surgery has been shown to result in poorer postoperative range of motion and decreased functional outcomes. Although the time frames vary across studies, surgery within 1 week of injury seems to be associated with improved outcomes.

Other preoperative factors that correlate with a poor result are preoperative neurologic deficit, a history of cigarette smoking, excesve alcohol consumption, and female sex. Poorer results associated with the latter are somewhat controversial because in the studies that identified ths finding, women were significantly older than men, which is a significant confounding variable.

Tuberosity position and healing may be the most important factors in determining outcome. Greater tuberosity malunion is the most common complication associated with hemiarthroplasty for four-part proximal humerus fractures. Final tuberosity position of more than 5 mm above or more than 10 mm below the prosthetic head is associated with poor results. A final position of more than 2 cm below the prosthetic humeral head also has been associated with a poor functional result. The best range of motion has been reported to occur if the tuberosity is between 10 and 16 mm below the humeral head. Although these results differ somewhat, a nonanatomic final positiion of the tuberosity generally is believed to interfere with rotator cuff function and compromise range of motion and function. Lesser tuberosity malunion has received much less attention as a factir affecting outcome and does not appear to be as significant as greater tuberosity position (Zuckerman & Sajadi 2007).

Studying the clinical and radiologic parameters that can explain unsatisfactory results, final tuberosity malposition correlates with unsatisfactory results as well as superior migration of the prosthesis, poor position of the greater tuberosity and women over age 75 years (likely with osteopenic bone) (Boileau et al 2002).

At least five compelling reasons exist to reattach the tuberosities and obtain bone healing when performing a reverse shoulder prosthesis: 1) humeral length is restored and thus the deltoid is tensioned optimally; 2) joint stability is improved as a function of the restored humeral length and reconstructed anterior and posterior soft tissue walls; 3) the risk of of infection is reduced as the subacromial dead-space is minimised and the surrounding soft-tissues are better vascularised. 4) better primary implant stability reduces the probability of humeral implant loosening and 5) active (specifically external) rotation is restored, crucial for activities of daily living in elderly patients (Boileau et al 2010).

3.4 Avoiding pitfalls and complications

Complications following hemiarthroplasty for acute proximal humerus fractures include infection, neurologic injury, preiprosthetic fracture, instability, tuberosity malunion and nonunion, rotator cuff tear, heterotopic ossification, glenoid erosion, and stiffness. Although the incidence of any specific complication is relatively low, the cumulative incidence represents at least 15%.

The incience of infection and wound healing problems is about 4% and includes acute postoperative infections and subacute delayed presentations within 6 months of the procedure. Factors that increase the risk of infection include the need for a second operation performed within a short period of time and a compromise immune system. Preventing infection requires meticulous attention to surgical preparation and drapping, particularly because of the potential contamination from the axilla. Perioperative antibiotics are indicated. Meticulous handling of soft tissues also is important. The fact that these injures occur more commonly in enderly patients whose tissues are more sensitive to injury and surgery further emphasizes its importance. If wound problems develop early in the postoperative course, treatment should be aggresive, including additional antibiotics and surgical debridement, if necessary (Young et al 2010).

Instability following hemiarthroplasty also can be a significant problem. The definition of instability varies widely, which affects the reported incidence of this problem. Several factors predispose patients to the development of instability, including component malposition, rotator cuff compromise, and tuberosity problems. Of these, component malposition is a critically important predisposing factor. Instability may result if the humeral component is placed too high or too low, resulting in secondary impingement or poor soft-tissue tension, respectively. Improper placement of the component in excessive anteversion or retroversion may lead to dislocation and tuberosity failure (Voos et al 2010).

If the component is placed in an incorrect amount of version or if humeral length is not properly restored, the risk of instability is greater. Careful attention to positioning the component intraoperatively and managing that position during cementing is essential. Inserting the component in proper version requires the use of consistent landmarks. Obtaining proper version and length during cementing can be difficult; therefore, we find the use of intraoperative fracture jigs to be beneficial. Component malposition can be prevented if a reliable method to obtain and mantain malposition during insertion is used. We believe that cemented fixation of these components is mandatory to mantain position, particularly in the absense of mataphyseal bony support (Young et al 2010).

The so-called "unhappy triad," involves prosthesis with excessive height and retroversion and the greater tuberosity is positioned too low. This combination was frequently associated with poor functional results and persistent pain and stiffness. Studies have also demonstrated that acute reconstruction (less than four weeks after the injury) results in better functional outcomes because of the ease of tuberosity reconstruction (Boileau et al 2000).

Rotator cuff compromise also causes instablity and usually develops as a result of tuberosity compromise. Preventing this problem requires secure fixation and proper positioning of the tuberosity. If the tuberosity becomes detached, particularly in the early postoperative period, instability often can result. Detachment of the lesser tuberosity compromises anterior support and can result in anterior instability (Young et al 2010).

Detachment of the greater tuberosity can result in significant superior and anterior instability. Although posterior instability can occur, it is less common. Factors that predispose patients to tuberosity detachment are inadequate tuberosity fixation and noncompliance with the postoperative rehabilitation. Secure tuberosity fixation and reattachment using the priciples (transverse, longitudinal, and cerclage fixation) will decrease the risk of fixation failure. A supervised, structured rehabilitaion program also can limit the potential for patient noncompliance. The treatment of instability following tuberosity failure can be difficult. If detachment is identified early, reattachment should be considered. Tuberositiy detachment identified more than 6 months after surgery is more probelmatic. Mobilization and attachment of tuberosities can be quite difficult at this time. If the patient reports significant pain and demonstrates instability, the revision surgery, possibly to a reverse shoulder arthroplasty, may be necessary.

Tuberosity nonunion is another significant complication following hemiarthroplasty. The factors that predispose patients to nonunion are related to the method of reattachment, particularly the ability to obtain proper reduction and secure fixation. The quality of bone and soft tissue also affect fixation. The significance of tuberosity nonunion can vary, but generally relates to the degree of migration and displacement. Limited amounts of migration and displacement frequently result in weakness and limited motion but not instability. With significant displacement, the patient will demonstrate weakness and limited motion, as well as instability and pain. The best approach to prevent tuberosity nonunion is use of an optimal method of reattachment.

Malunion of the greater or lesser tuberosity can occur, although probably with less frequency than nonunion. Malunion usually occurs as a result of either inadequate reduction at the time of surgery or inadequate fixation, which allows migration of the fragment with healing into a malunited position. Thus, proper positioning of the tuberosity intraoperatively is mandatory to avoid these problems. If necessary, intraoperative radiographs should be obtained to confirm the position. Radiographs also should be obtained early in the postoperative period to ensure that migration has not occurred. Malunion of the greater tuberosity is a much more significant problem than that of the lesser tuberosity. Posterior or superior displacement of the greater tuberosity restricts motion and can be a source of pain. Treatment of tuberosity malunion depends on functional significance. If significant pain and limited motion can be attributed to tuberosity malunion, surgical management consisting of osteotomy, mobilization, and reattachment to a more anatomic position can be considered. If the component is not in an optimal position, the component revision may be necessary. These procedures tend to be difficult and, clearly, the most effective treatment of tuberosity malunion is prevention.

Heterotopic ossification following hemiarthroplasty for acute fractures is relatively common, although it generally is not clinically significant. Small areas of heterotopic ossification an reactive bone can develop, but these generally do not interfere with function or compromise outcomes. However, more extensive ossification, particularly in the subacromial space, or bone bridging from the acromion to the proximal humerus can be significant. The factors that predispose to clinically heterotopic ossification include high-energy injuries (fracture-dislocations) and delays in surgery longer than 10 to 14 days after the acute injury. Heterotopic ossification also can develop when the procedure is performed after an early failure of internal fixation. The second procedure, particularly when it is performed 2 to 4 weeks after the initial procedure, carries a signinficant increased risk of heterotopic ossification. Whenever possible, it is important to take measures to prevent the formation of heterotopic bone. At the time of the initial surgery, meticulous technique to minimize soft-tissue trauma is important. The timing of surgery also is important. Whenever possible, the "at risk" period should be avoided. For those patients who are felt to be at high risk for heterotopic bone development, prophylactic measures can be considered, including anti-inlammatory medications postoperatively and/or the use of single-dose radiation therapy. The use of preventive measures has to be balanced with the potential to interfer with tuberosity healing and should be individualized for each patient (Young et al 2010).

Plausinis et al reported the complicationes that took place after humeral head replacement and included infection, neurologic injury, intraoperative fracture, instability, tuberosity malunion and nonunion, rotator cuff tear, heterotopic ossification, glenoid erosion, and stiffness. When technical factors such as tuberosity malunion or component malpositioning are considered as postoperative complications, the incidence of complications is relatively high (Plausinis et al 2005).

Cazeneuve et al described the clinical and radiological outcome of 36 fractures at a mean of 6.6 years (1 to 16) in which the mean Constant score was 58.5 and was reduced to 53 points with the further follow-up. A total of 23 patients (63%) had radiological evidence of loosening of the glenoid component. Nevertheless, only one patient had aseptic loosening of the baseplate at 12 years' follow-up (Cazeneuve et al 2010).

Wall et al reported a series of 186 with 191 retained reverse total shoulder arthroplasty prostheses who were followed for an average of 39.9 months. Overall, the average Constant score improved from 23 points before surgery to 60 points at the time of follow-up and 173 of the 186 patients were satisfied or very satisfied with the result. Dislocation (fifteen cases) and infection (eight cases) were the most common complications among the 199 shoulders that were followed for two years or were revised prior to the minimum two-year follow-up. Patients who received the reverse prosthesis at the time of a revision arthroplasty had a higher complication rate than did those who received the reverse prosthesis at the time of a primary arthroplasty. The most common complications were dislocation (fifteen cases; prevalence, 7.5%) and infection (eight cases; prevalence, 4.0%). Glenoid fractures, postoperative humeral fractures, symptomatic hardware, musculocutaneous nerve palsy, radial nerve palsy, glenoid sphere loosening, and glenoid base loosening also occurred in five or fewer cases each (Wall & Walch 2007).

To evaluate functional outcome after hemiarthroplasty for displaced proximal humeral fractures and to review whether prosthesis type, intraoperative technique or previous ipsilateral shoulder surgery could affect the outcome, Fallatah et al reviewed the medical records and radiographs of patients who had undergone hemiarthroplasty for proximal humeral fractures between 1992 and 2000. They concluded that soft tissue status and operative technique played an important role in late postoperative pain and range of motion. Hemiarthroplasty after failed open reduction and internal fixation is associated with inferior results (Fallatah et al 2008).

In the retrospective study of Gallinet D et al, forty patients were treated by shoulder replacement for three- or four-part displaced fractures of the proximal humerus between 1996 and 2004. Twenty-one had a hemiarthroplasty and 19 were treated by reverse prosthesis. The reverse prosthesis group showed better results in terms of abduction, anterior elevation and Constant score. Rotation was better in the hemiarthroplasty group. They concluded that in three- or four-part displaced proximal humerus fracture, arthroplasty did not ensure recovery of pretrauma shoulder function. Management is therefore to be decided in terms of outcome predictability and rapid recovery of daily comfort for elderly patients (Gallinet et al 2009).

Hemiarthroplasty can provide good functional results, but depends on tuberosity union quality and this often necessitates a prolonged immobilization. Reverse prostheses provide reliable, rapid and predictable results in terms of abduction, anterior elevation and pain relief, but impaired rotation; this impacts quality of life and long-term implant durability (glenoid notching).

Reverse prostheses should thus prove advantageous in the treatment of complex fractures of the proximal humerus if these two drawbacks can be resolved and at present seem indicated on condition that the patient is no younger than 70 years of age (Gallinet et al 2009).

Compito et al reviewed the important factors for a successful outcome, including gentle soft tissue technique, secure placement of the prosthesis with proper version and height, secure tuberosity reconstruction, meticulous rotator cuff repair, and a motivated patient who is able to understand and perform the rigorous postoperative rehabilitation. Unsatisfactory results are associated with tuberosity detachment, prosthetic loosening, inadequate or noncompliant rehabilitation, preoperative nerve injury, humeral malposition, dislocation, deep infection, and ectopic hone formation (Compito et al 1994).

On the basis of the current literature, Voos et al list arthroplasties for the treatment of complex proximal humeral fractures in descending order with regard to their clinical success as follows: (1) hemiarthroplasty in a patient with reconstructible tuberosities, (2) reverse total shoulder arthroplasty in a patient with reconstructible tuberosities, (3) reverse total shoulder arthroplasty in a patient without reconstructible tuberosities, and (4) hemiarthroplasty in a patient without reconstructible tuberosities (Voos et al 2010).

This review covers the indications, technique, results, and complications associated with the use of prostheses for proximal humeral fractures. Meticulous technique, especially in regards to tuberosity fixation, is necessary for successful reconstruction. The use of the Reverse Total Shoulder prosthesis is in evolution but does offer exciting options in the management of these difficult patients (Voos et al 2010).

4. References

[1] Antuña SA, Sperling JW, Cofield RH. Shoulder hemiarthroplasty for acute fractures of the proximal humerus: a minimum five-year follow-up. J Shoulder Elbow Surg. 2008;17(2):202-9.

[2] Bastian JD, Hertel R. Osteosynthesis and hemiarthroplasty of fractures of the proximal humerus: Outcomes in a consecutive case series. J Shoulder Elbow Surg 2009;19:216-219.

[3] Bigliani LU. Fractures of the proximal humerus. In: Rockwood CA, Green DP, eds. Fractures in Adults. 3rd ed. Philadelphia, Pa: JB Lippincott Completed/mh; 1990:871-927.

[4] Boileau P, Krishnan SG, Tinsi L, et al. Tuberosity malposition and migration: Reasons for poor outcomes after hemiarthroplasty fro displaced fractures of the proximal humerus. J Shoulder Elbow Surg 2002;11(5): 401-412.

[5] Boileau P, Trojani C, Walch G, Krishnan SG, Romeo A, Sinnerton R. Shoulder arthroplasty for the treatment of the sequelae of fractures of the proximal humerus. J Shoulder Elbow Surg 2001;10:299-308.

[6] Boileau P, Walch G, Krishnan SG. Tuberosity osteosynthesis and hemiarthoplasty for four-part fractures of the proximal humerus. Tech Shoulder Elbow Surg 2000;1:96-109.

[7] Boileau P, Moineau N, Brassart, Clavert, Favard L, Sirveaux F, O'Shea K. Reverse Shoulder Fracture-Prosthesis for the treatment of proximal humeral fractures in elderly patients. Shoulder Concepts 2010:231-43.

[8] Bufquin T, Hersan A, Hubert L, Massin P. Reverse shoulder arthroplasty for the treatment of three- and four-part fractures of the proximal humerus in the elderly: a prospective review of 43 cases with a short-term follow-up. J Bone Joint Surg. 2007 Apr;89(4):516-20.

[9] Cazeneuve JF, Cristofari DJ. The reverse shoulder prosthesis in the treatment of fractures of the proximal humerus in the elderly. J Bone Joint Surg. 2010;92(4):535-9.

[10] Compito CA, Self EB, Bigliani LU. Arthroplasty and acute shoulder trauma. Reasons for success and failure. Clin Orthop 1994;307:27-36.

[11] Demirhan M, Kilicoglu O, Altinel L, Eralp L, Akalin Y. Prognostic factors in prosthetic replacement for acute proximal humerus fractures. J Orthop Trauma 2003;17(3):181-189.

[12] Duralde XA, Leddy LR. The results of ORIF of displaced unstable proximal humeral fractures using a locking plate. J Shoulder Elbow Surg 2010;19:480-488.

[13] Esen E, Dogramaci Y, Gultekin S, Deveci MA, et al. Factors affecting results of patients with humeral proximal end fractures undergoing primary hemiarthroplasty: A restrospective study in 42 patients. Injury 2009;40:1336-1341.

[14] Fallatah S, Dervin GF, Brunet JA, Conway AF, Hrushowy H. Functional outcome after proximal humeral fractures treated with hemiarthroplasty. Can J Surg. 2008;51(5):361-5.

[15] Flatow EL, Bigliani LU. Locating and protecting the axillary nerve in the shoulder surgery; the Tug Test. Orthop Rev. 1992;21:503-505.

[16] Frankle M, Siegal S, Pupello D, et al. The reverse shoulder prosthesis for glenohumeral arthritis associated with severe rotator cuff deficiency. A minimum two-year follow-up study of sixty patients. J Bone Joint Surg Am 2005;87(8):1697-1705.

[17] Frankle MA, Ondrovic LE, Markee BA, Harris ML, Lee WE 3rd. Stability of tuberosity reattachment in proximal humeral hemiarthroplasty. J Shoulder Elbow Surg 2002;11(5):413-420.

[18] Frankle MA, Greenwald DP, Markee BA, Ondrovic LE, Lee WE 3rd. Biomechanical effects of malposition of tuberosity fragments on the humeral prosthetic reconstruction for four-part proximal humerus fractures. J Shoulder Elbow Surg 2001;10(4):321-326.

[19] Gallinet D, Clappaz P, Garbuio P, Tropet Y, Obert L. Three or four parts complex proximal humerus fractures: hemiarthroplasty versus reverse prosthesis: a comparative study of 40 cases. Orthop Traumatol Surg Res. 2009 Feb;95(1):48-55.

[20] Goldman RT, Koval KJ, Cuomo F, et al. Functional outcomes after humeral head replacement for acute three and four-part proximal humerus fractures. J Shoulder Elbow Surg 1995;4:81-86.

[21] Green A, Bamard L, Limbrid RS. Humeral head replacement for acute, four-part proximal humerus fractures. J Shoulder Elbow Surg 1993;2:249-254.

[22] Hawkins RJ, Switlyk P. Acute prosthetic replacement for severe fractures of the proximal humerus. Clin Orthop 1993;289:156-160.

[23] 23 Huffman GR, Itamura JM, McGarry MH, Duong L, et al. Neer Award 2006: Biomechanical assessment of inferior tuberosity placement during hemiarthroplasty for four-part proximal humeral fractures. J Shoulder Elbow Surg 2008;17(2):189-196.

[24] Jaberg H, Warner JJ, Jakob RP. Percutaneous stabilization of unstable fractures of the humerus. J Bone Joint SUrg Am 1992;74:508-515.

[25] Kontakis G, Koutras C. Tosounidis T, Giannoudis P. Early management of proximal humeral fractures with hemiarthroplasty. J Bone Joint Surg (Br) 2008;90B(11):1407-1413.

[26] Lervick GN, Carroll RM, Levine WN. Complications after hemiarthroplasty for fractures of the proximal humerus. Instr Course Lect. 2003;52:3-12.

[27] Levine WN, Connor PM, Yamaguchi K, Self EB, et al. Humeral head replacement for proximal humeral fractures. Orthopedics 1998;21(1):68-73.

[28] Martin TG, Iannotti JP. Reverse total shoulder arthroplasty for acute fractures and failed management after proximal humeral fractures. Orthop Clin North Am. 2008;39(4):451-7.

[29] Mighell MA, Kolm GP, Colinge CA, Frankle MA. Outcomes of hemiarthroplasty for fractures of the proximal humerus. J Shoulder Elbow Surg 2003;12:569-577.

[30] Moeckel BH, Dines DM, Warren RF, Altchek DW. Modular hemiarthroplasty for fractures of the proximal part of the humerus. J Bone Joint Surg Am 1992;74:884-889.

[31] Murachovsky J, Ikemoto RY, Nascimento LG, Milani C, Warner JJ. Pectoralis major tendon reference (PMT): A new method for accurate restoration of humeral length with hemiarthroplasty for fracture. J Shoulder Elbow Surg 2006;15(6):675-678.

[32] Neer CS. Fractures. In: Shoulder Reconstruction. Philadelphia, PA: WB Saunders Co. 1990:363-420.

[33] Neer CS. Displaced proximal humeral fractures, I: classification and evaluation. J Bone Joint Surg Am 1970;52:1077-1089.

[34] Neer CS. Displaced proximal humeral fractures, II: treatment of three-part and four-part displacement. J Bone Joint Surg Am 1970;52:1090-1103.

[35] Pijls BGCW, Werner PH, Eggen PJ. Alternative humeral tubercle fixation in shoulder hemiarthroplasty for fractures of the proximal humerus. J Shoulder Elbow Surg 2010;19:282-289.

[36] Plausins D, Kwon YW, Zuckerman JD. Complications of humeral head replacement for proximal humeral fractures. AAOS Instruc Course 2005;54:371-380.

[37] Reuther F, Mühlhäusler B, Wahl D, Nijs S. Functional outcome of shoulder hemiarthroplasty for fractures: A multicentre analysis. Injury. 2010;41(6):606-12.

[38] Robinson CM, Page RS, Hill RMF, Sanders DL, et al. Primary hemiarthroplasty for treatment of proximal humeral fractures. J Bone Joint Surg 2003;85A (7):1215-1223.

[39] Shrader MW, Sanchez-Sotelo J, Sperling JW, et al. Understanding proximal humerus fractures: image analysis, classification, and treatment. J Shoulder Elbow Surg 2005; 14(5): 497-505.

[40] Tanner MW, Cofield RH. Prosthetic arthroplasty for fractures and fracture-dislocations of the proximal humerus. Clin Orthop 1983;179:116-128.

[41] Voos JE, Dines JS, Dines DM. Arthroplasty for fractures of the proximal part of the humerus. J Bone Joint Surg Am. 2010 Jun;92(6):1560-7.

[42] Wall B, Walch G. Reverse Shoulder Arthroplasty for the Treatment of Proximal Humeral Fractures. Hand Clin 23,2007:425-430.

[43] Young TB, Wallace WA. Conservative treatment of fractures and fracture-dislocations of the upper end of the humerus. J Bone Joint Surg Br 1985;67:373-377.

[44] Zyto K. Non-operative treatment of comminuted fractures of the proximal humerus in elderly patients. Injury 1998;29(5):349-352.

[45] Young SW, Segal BS, Turner PC, Poon PC. Comparison of functional outcomes of reverse shoulder arthroplasty versus hemiarthroplasty in the primary treatment of acute proximal humerus fracture. ANZ J Surg. 2010;80(11):789-93.

[46] Zuckerman JD, Sajadi KR. Proximal Humerus Fractures: Hemiarthroplasty for Four-Part Fractures. Advanced Reconstruction Shoulder. AAOS 2007:30:283-98.

8

Postoperative Therapy for Metacarpophalangeal Arthroplasty

Nicola Massy-Westropp
School of Health Sciences, University of South Australia
Australia

1. Introduction

Since the earliest metacarpophalangeal (MCP) arthroplasties in the 1950s, numerous resurfacing and excisional arthroplasties, and a greater choice of surgical tools and techniques to implant the prostheses have become available. Of the excisional arthroplasties, one-piece and two-piece hinge designs, constrained by screws or unconstrained, cemented and non-cemented, have been designed (1) Surgeons now perform these procedures as day surgery, and leave as much original bone as possible in the likelihood of replacing the prosthesis as the patient ages.

At the time of surgery, synovectomy and soft-tissue balancing procedures are often performed to increase lateral joint stability or enhance the biomechanical advantage of the tendons around the operated joint. These procedures may necessitate post-operative immobilisation, specific joint positioning and strict motion protocols to achieve the best soft tissue range of motion and stability around the prosthesis (2-6).

The efficacy of postoperative therapy regimens also requires research, as they affect patient outcome, and are time-consuming and expensive. The aim of this review is to determine which postoperative regimen are most effective in achieving freedom from pain and function, and if any particular regimen is best suited to a specific prosthesis or soft-tissue balancing procedure at the time of surgery.

2. Method

For inclusion in this review, studies had to evaluate the efficacy of a post-arthroplasty regimen for patients who had metacarpophalangeal or joint arthroplasty. Preferred study designs were metanalyses, systematic reviews, and randomised controlled trials, but all published literature except expert opinion was accepted. Patients may have received any type of implant and soft-tissue procedure, due to rheumatoid arthritis, osteoarthritis or trauma.

Electronic databases searched were the Cochrane Musculoskeletal Disease Group Register, The Cochrane Library of Systematic review, Google Scholar, and Scopus. Manual searches included of the Journal of Hand Therapy, Hand Therapy and the Journal of Arthroplasty. Search terms in all combinations included 'joint replacement, hand, wrist metacarpophalangeal, arthroplasty, rehabilitation, post-operative, occupational therapy, physical therapy'. The search included papers from 1990 onward, aiming to find research about currently used prostheses and not prostheses of older designs and materials.

Studies were appraised as described by the Cochrane Collaboration (7) for sources of methodological bias that could decrease the internal validity of a study. The types of methodological bias were in patient selection, equality of treatment, attrition of patients, and detection of all relevant outcomes. If the study could not be fully appraised from the publication, information was sought by writing to the authors.

3. Results

Sixteen studies described post-operative therapy for MCP joint replacement in enough detail to understand the treatment schedule. Four hundred and twenty-seven patients in these studies had rheumatoid arthritis, 19 had osteoarthritis and one had psoriatic arthritis. There were four randomised trials (one about post-operative therapy), three prospective cohort studies, three prospective case series (two about post-operative therapy), one case study about post-operative therapy, and the remaining were retrospective case series. Missing data was obtained from two authors, to assist in reviewing the rigour of the studies, but many authors could not be contacted.

The randomised controlled trial study found to specifically compare post-operative regimes for metacarpophalangeal arthroplasty (8) randomised patients into postoperative therapy groups that both included dynamic splinting, but the treatment group also included continuous passive motion. These researchers found no difference between treatment groups. Thomsen, Boeckstyns and Leth-Espensen(2003) (9) and retrospectively reviewed consecutive patients who had either dynamic MCP extension splinting, or had static splinting that was removed for exercises post-operatively. They found that residual extension lag was significantly less (p = 0.002) in the dynamically-splinted group, concluding that postoperative dynamic splinting was useful. Groth, Watkins and Paynter, (1996)(10) retrospectively compared patients who had dynamic flexion with those who had dynamic extension splinting, and found that those who had post-operative dynamic flexion splinting had greater post-operative MCP flexion. Burr, Pratt and Smith (2002)(11), Burr and Pratt (1999)(12) focussed their research on post-operative therapy, but neither study had a comparison treatment group. No further studies compared post-operative treatment regimes, therefore the results of the remaining studies can only be appreciated as a combination of surgery, implant and post-operative therapy.

One outcome common to nearly all postoperative patients in every study was the relief of pain once the diseased joint had been removed by surgery. Negative outcomes such as wound infection, implant loosening and migration were reported, in small proportions. Compliance with splinting and therapy was not discussed. Sixteen studies described the outcome of different implants and postoperative therapy regimes for MCP arthroplasty.

Features common to many regimens (Table 1) were postoperative avoidance of any hand activity for the first three to six weeks and long-term avoidance of ulnar forces on the fingers. Nearly all regimens began between the second and seventh postoperative day.

Regimens could be divided into two main categories with regard to splinting and exercise. Static splint regimens involved removal of the splint for active MCP range of motion exercises, and dynamic splint regimens involved active-assisted MCP extension and active MCP flexion exercises within the splint.

STUDY AND DESIGN	PARTICIPANTS	TREATMENT	OUTCOME	POTENTIAL FOR BIAS
Escott, Ronald, Judd and Bogoch 2010(13) Prospective cohort	N=33 with RA MCP flexion mean 89-91° extension lag mean 61-65°.	Treatment groups had Neuflex or Swanson joint prostheses. Day 4-6 Resting Splint, neutral wrist, 40° MCP flexion, 10-20° Week 1-3 MCP AROM flexion and extension and PROM for wrist and IP Patients were instructed to remove the splint only for ROM exercises during the next 3/52 3/52 PROM MCP flexion and extension of joints 4/52, splint removal for light ADL and ROM Splint wear at times of risk and at night. 6/52 splint at night only, and strengthening initiated Night splinting to minimum of 3/12 Patients educated to avoid positions of deformity.	One Year Outcomes: Both group showed significant improvement in mean Sollerman score and all 6 MHQ domains (p=.001), and MCP extension (mean ROM not provided) Both groups showed significant increases in grip strength improved significantly at the larger Jamar grip position 4 but not smaller positions 2&3 No significant differences between treatment groups, except those with Swanson implants demonstrated higher Michigan Hand Outcomes Questionnaire scores.	Patient selection included highly variable patients Detection of outcome may be inadequate at one year. Detection of outcome may not be powered Detection suffers from no comparison group
Harada, Okumura and Takahashi 2010(14) Retrospective case series	11 patients with RA mean AROM MP 52/95 Mean grip 5.1 kg	Patients had Swanson or Avanta silicone implants. Day 4-5: An outrigger splint was used for MPJ extension. Rubber band was pulled on an angle toward the radial-sided finger. Active flexion and passive extension of MPJ on the outrigger splint was started. 2/52 An outrigger splint was added for MP flexion. Outrigger splints for MP flexion and extension were used alternately every hour and alternately each night. 3-4 /52: Active and gentle passive motion of MPJ. 6 /52: Use of hand in light ADL.	mean follow-up 8.7/12 (4-14) mean AROM MP 5/65 Mean grip 4.9 kg	Patient selection included highly variable patients Detection of outcome may be inadequate at one year. Detection of outcome may not be powered Detection suffers from no comparison group Attrition of patients from series
Chung, Burns, Wilgis, Burke, Regan, Kim and Fox 2009,(15) Prospective cohort	N=70 with RA Michigan Hand Outcome Questionnaire mean score =37/100 (18) Grip=5.7(6) Key Pinch=3.5(2)	Patients had Swanson implants. Day 5-7 Dynamic MCP extension splint all times for 6/52 6/52 light ADL, splint worn in evening only 12/52 splint is discharged, normal ADL allowed.	One Year Outcomes: Michigan Hand Outcome Questionnaire mean score =59/100 (22) Grip=6.2(5) Key Pinch=3.1(2)	Patient selection included highly variable patients Detection of outcome may be inadequate at one year. Detection suffers from no comparison group

STUDY AND DESIGN	PARTICIPANTS	TREATMENT	OUTCOME	POTENTIAL FOR BIAS
Pettersson, Wagnsjo, Hulin 2006(16) Randomised trial	N=40 with RA Mean pain 3.5-4.5/10 Mean extension deficit 51-53° Mean MCP arc of motion = 33°	Patients randomly allocated to have NeuFlex or Sutter implants. Day 0-5 hand immobilised in plaster, only PIP joints free. Day 5 active mobilisation was started 3-5/24. Static splint allowed full PIP ROM, restricted MCP 0- 20°and stabilised the MCP in radial and ulnar deviation and gave volar support for t MCPs 6/52 splint replaced by night extension splint used for the first year to prevent ulnar deviation. Gradually increased motion initiated without radial and ulnar pressure 8/52, daily activities without weight bearing in ulnar direction were allowed. 3/12, no restriction except for ADL or work.	One Year Outcomes Mean pain 2.8-3.5/10 Mean extension deficit 20-21° Mean MCP arc of motion =49°	Patient selection included highly variable patients Detection of outcome may be inadequate at one year. Detection suffers from no comparison group
Nunez and Citron, 2005(17) Case series (uncertain if prospective)	N=seven patients, 10 implants with OA Mean pain = 68%, mean MCP arc of motion = 43°, patient-perceived strength 31%, patient-perceived satisfaction 44%	Patients had Ascension two piece unconstrained prosthesis. First 48 hours Patient asked to flex fingers in post-operative dressing After 48 hours, dressings are removed and patients may use passive assistance to achieve full ROM as soon as possible.	Follow-up one to four years one patient had a slight temporary wound inflammation Mean pain = 3%, mean MCP arc of motion = 52°, patient-perceived strength 86%, patient-perceived satisfaction 93%	Detection of outcome may be inadequate at one year. Detection of outcome may not be powered Detection suffers from no comparison group
Rettig, Luca and Murphy 2005(18) Retrospective case series	N=12 with OA Metacarpophalangeal joint flexion was 53° no excessive MCP ulnar deviation	Patients received Swanson implants, some had grommets over their implants. Day 0 to 3-7 Patients were placed in a bulky wrist, MCP PIP immobilization splint Day 3-7Gentle active extension and flexion commenced Until 6-8/52 night, static extension splint. 4/52 strengthening program.	6-8/52 MCP flexion 59° Nine patients noted excellent overall improvement, three said good overall improvement Nine patients stated excellent pain relief, one patient had good pain relief, and two had satisfactory pain relief. Nine patients 9 reported functional improvement > 75% Seven patients were able to perform the Jebsen-Taylor functional assessment within the normal time.	Detection of outcome may be inadequate at one year. Detection of outcome Nine may not be powered

STUDY AND DESIGN	PARTICIPANTS	TREATMENT	OUTCOME	POTENTIAL FOR BIAS
Moller, Sollerman Geirjer, Kopylov and Tagil 2005(19) Randomised trial	N=30 with RA, one psoriatic arthritis Active ROM =32° (range 8–58°) This was assumed to be MCP flexion. Mean MCP Extension deficit= 42-47 (2-86)	Patients randomised to Swanson or Avanta implants Day-7 hand mobilized in a dynamic extension splint, aiming to achieve 45° flexion. Night static palmar splint with MCP slightly flexed. PIP extension splint used if there was tendency to flex PIPs instead of MCPs. 4 /52goal was 70° flexion. If flexion was restricted, a dynamic flexion splint was used. 6/52 light loading permitted, dynamic extension splint weaned 12/52 Splints discharged and loading as permitted by pain.	Two year follow-up Active ROM improved to 42°(range 20–60°) after surgery (p= 0.04) in the Avanta group, whereas no significant improvement was seen in the Swanson Mean MCP Extension deficit= 16-19 (1-43)	Patient selection included highly variable patients no Detection suffers from no therapy comparison group. group
Parkkila, Belt, Hakala, Kautiainen and Leppolahti 2005(20) Randomised trial	N=53 patients with RA, 58 hands operated.	Patients randomised to receive Sutter or Swanson prostheses. All received physiotherapy for 2/12, seven having continuous passive motion in and out of hospital. 2/12 five patients had finger manipulation if they were stiff.	Four – Five year follow-up Five patients died, one was lost and two had strokes. Six patients (three from each group) had revision surgery. More patients showed osteolysis around the implant, if they had Sutter implants, over Swanson implants.	Patient selection included highly variable patients Attrition of patients Detection suffers from no therapy comparison group
Thomsen, Boeckstyns and Leth-Espensen 2003(21) Retrospective case series	N=22 Pre-operative measures not available	Patients received Swanson implants. Group 1 Dynamic splint. Day 6-4/52 dynamic extension and radial deviation splint used continuously active assisted flexion and passive extension exercises encouraged during the same period. Patients attended physiotherapy 3-5/7. Week 4-6/52 dynamic splint was night only Group 2 No dynamic splint Day 0-5/7static splinting, exercises as described above were encouraged without the splint, static splint retained between exercises. 2/52 day time static splinting discontinued 2-4/52 night static splinting	Group 1 Dynamic splint(n = 41) nearly 5 years follow up Extension lag 10 (0–50) Flexion 60 (5–90) Range of movement 45 (5–80) Ulnar deviation 10 (0–30) Group 2 No dynamic splint (n = 29) nearly 2 years follow up Extension lag 20 (0–45)* Flexion 60 (30–80) Ulnar deviation 10 (0–20) * $p = 0.002$	Patient selection may have included highly variable patients–no data Detection of difference in outcome may not be powered Attrition of patients high from both groups

STUDY AND DESIGN	PARTICIPANTS	TREATMENT	OUTCOME	POTENTIAL FOR BIAS
Radmer, Andresen and Sparman 2003 (22) Prospective Case series	N=eight women with RA marked ulnar deviation. mean active flexion = 30 (15-40°) mean extensor lag 55° (40-100°).	Patients received WEKO hinged implants Day 0 - 2or 3 hand immobilized in palmar forearm plaster splint Day 2-3 - 6/52 dynamic splint. Position not described Exercises for the fingers were performed out of the splint, without restriction. Exercises not described.	One Year Outcomes: 20/28 prostheses had migrated mean active flexion = 30(22-35°) mean extensor lag 42° (40-48°). average ulnar deviation 20° (0-50)°	Detection of outcome may be inadequate at one year. Detection of outcome may not be powered Detection suffers from no comparison group
Ishikawa, Murasawa and Hanyu 2002(23) Retrospective case series	N=64 with RA, 20 implants into the thumbs Mean MCP flexion=72-73° Mean MCP extension lag=35-39° Pain=23-28/100	Patients received Swanson implants, some had grommets over their implants. Those with thumb implants received a 'flexible hinge toe implant'. Day0-5 a 'short arm splint' was worn Day 5 - 6/52 dynamic splint (assumed to be MCP extension) with AROM and PROM of MCP joints	Mean follow-up six years 12 revision surgeries Mean MCP flexion= 49-50° Mean MCP extension lag=15-28 Pain=0-6/100	Patient selection included highly variable patients Attrition of patients from series Detection suffers from no therapy comparison group
Burr, Pratt and Smith, 2002 (11) Prospective Case series	n = 15 with RA	Swanson prostheses Day 5-7 - 4/52:Two static splints, alternated 24 hourly, with MCP at 0° in one splint, and 60°	Mean MCP flexion unchanged; improvements in pain, MCP extension, and power grip	Detection suffers from no therapy comparison group
Burr and Pratt, 1999 (12) Case study	n = One patient with RA	flexion in the other. No ADL 3/52 biofeedback to finger flexors and extensors no heavy lifting 4/52 IP ROM, MCP flexion, RD 3-10x hourly, 4/52 Light ADL 8/52 normal ADL 12/52 return to work, heavy lifting	At 8/52 0-15° MCP extension and 60-70° MCP flexion at 8/52.	ncies of studies reporting inadequate at 8/52
Ring, Simmons and Hayes, 1998 (8) RCT	n = 25 with RA	"Silicone arthroplasty" Day 2-7 Dynamic MCP extension splint with RD, until 6/52 Night MCP 0° for 12/52 MCP and IP ROM 3.10 every hour 2 hours in splint; RD at 4/52 Treatment group IP ROM, received MCP CPM No pinch for 12/52	at 5/12 CPM group did not achieve significant increases in ROM or strength	Detection of outcome may be inadequate at 5/12 Detection suffers from no therapy comparison group

STUDY AND DESIGN	PARTICIPANTS	TREATMENT	OUTCOME	POTENTIAL FOR BIAS
Groth, Watkins and Paynter, 1996 (10) Retrospective case series	n = 34 patients, 46 hands with RA	Timing not recorded **Treatment group** Dynamic MCP flexion splint Night static splint, MCP 20–30° flexion	Uncertain of follow-up duration Treatment group had significantly more MCP flexion than cohort, but similar MCP extension	Patient selection may have included highly variable patients Selection of patients not described. Attrition of patients from both treatment groups
Stothard, Thompson and Sherris 1991 (Prospective cohort	N=25 patients with RA Mean ulnar deviation preoperatively 34°	Thirteen patients had Swanson MCP implants and crossed intrinsic transfer, 12 patients had MCP implant only. Day 3 static resting hand splint with high ulnar borders for all patients, removed four times daily for active radial deviation, flexion and extension. Day 8-10 PROM; no further details 3/52 splint worn at night only, light ADL 4/52 commenced occupational therapy; no further details	Follow-up 6-33/12 Five patients lost to follow-up Mean ulnar deviation 8° One infection occurred, one revision required Five patients in each treatment group had occasional pain or pain on use of their hand. Eighteen patients had improved or much improved function, three hand same function and three hand decreased function post-operatively. Crossed intrinsic transfer resulted in greater ROM	Patient selection included highly variable patients Detection of outcome may be inadequate at 6/12 Detection of outcome may not be powered Detection suffers from no therapy comparison group Attrition of patients from series

ADL=Activities of Daily Living, MCP= metacarpophalangeal, IP= interphalangeal joints; RD= radial deviation; RCT= randomized controlled trial; ROM= range of motion, RA=rheumatoid arthritis OA=osteoarthritis

Table 1. Studies reporting post-operative therapy for metacarpophalangeal arthroplasty, their design, treatment protocols, and outcomes.

4. Discussion

Sixteen studies described the outcome of different implants and postoperative therapy regimes for MCP arthroplasty. Two of these studies compared the efficacy of one regimen over another, one of these being prospective. Sambandam, Gul and Priyanka (2007)(25) state that 'most studies undermined the importance of this aspect (post-operative treatment) of the procedure' with regards to first carpometacarpal joint arthroplasty, but their claim could be expanded to arthroplasty of other joints of the hand. Post-operative protocols for splinting, activity and exercises are not always well-described, so although there were numerous studies about MCP arthroplasty, they are not included in this review.

Hand therapy for other conditions such as flexor tendon repair also offers multiple postoperative regimens. For example, healing tendons of the hand usually receive motion, but it may be passive, active, or a combination of all of these. The rationale for the various exercise regimens is based on biological healing of the tendon and the strength of the surgical repair, thus its ability to withstand stress without rupturing or gap formation (26,27). These patients usually have normal anatomy preoperatively, leaving few patient variables. Postoperative therapy regimens for MCP arthroplasty are also based on principles of healing and scar formation, but are not prescribed according to the patient's preoperative hand impairment, the type of implant used, or soft tissue balancing procedures performed. For example, patients having undergone extensor tendon rebalancing and recentralization may benefit from avoidance of passive flexion or avoidance of the extremes of flexion, much like a postoperative extensor tendon repair regime. The literature suggests that postoperative therapy for MCP arthroplasty has not been prescribed in this manner; rather, standard protocols have been designed and applied to consecutive patients.

To compare the efficacy of a new protocol, many patients would be required for allocation to various postoperative therapy groups. Their outcomes would have to be analyzed according to what protocol they received with the implant, surgery, and preoperative status as variables. The first difficulty in forming control or comparison groups lies in the infrequency of this procedure; for example Ring et al.(8) took three years to include 25 hands in their study.

The most common source of bias in the studies was selection bias, which occurs when patients are chosen for treatment or control groups as a result of characteristics that are expected to affect their outcome. Randomization is designed to control the confounding effects of differences between subjects at baseline, and the randomized trial is recommended as the best method of determining treatment efficacy. Here lies the second difficulty in forming control or comparison groups. Patients undergo MCP arthroplasty at all stages of their disease, evidenced by the wide range of motion deficits between the studies of Burr and Pratt, in which the case study patient had nearly normal preoperative MCP motion, and Burr et al., in which some patients had only 25° of MCP flexion, Measures of pain also varied widely in the latter study, ranging from "zero" to "eight out of ten." These baseline measurements demonstrate the difficulty in obtaining a homogeneous, comparable group of patients with rheumatoid arthritis.

The other three sources of bias described by the Cochrane Collaboration(7) were present in the reviewed studies. Performance bias occurs when patients receive a variation in duration, quality, or quantity of the treatment being studied, which was suspected in the continuous passive motion (CPM) study by Ring et al. Ring et al. describe the application of CPM in detail, except passive forces are described as "low" and treatment quantity is described as "as tolerated." As a result, the reader remains unsure of what amount of passive force is ineffective, as well as what quantity of treatment per day is ineffective.

Detection bias is determined if the timing of assessment, the outcome assessment used, or knowledge of the assessor of the patient's previous state could miss any relevant aspect of the outcome. This may have occurred in the study by Groth et al.,(10) in which some preoperative data were unavailable and patients were assessed at different postoperative time frames. Detection and comparison of outcomes between studies are only possible when the same outcome measures are used in a standardized manner. The researchers in this review all measured range of motion, but at different time frames (Table 1). Those who measured pain, cosmesis, and function applied different assessments at different time frames. The challenge of outcome measurement in rheumatology has led to the formation of focus groups such as OMERACT (Outcome Measures in Rheumatoid Arthritis Clinical Trials), who have made recommendations for outcome measures to be used in drug trials. OMERACT recommendations are not fully relevant to hand therapy research; however, the process of forming a focus group, and the development of assessment guidelines that allow comparison between homogeneous patients, is possible (28).

Attrition bias is determined if the loss of patients in the study is significant or varies between the treatment and control groups. This is common in long-term studies involving patients with rheumatoid arthritis, and was experienced by Groth et al.,(10) who were unable to obtain long-term follow-up of the patient group who received their extension protocol. Long-term follow-up is an issue with rheumatoid populations. These patients undergo numerous surgical and drug interventions, while their disease progresses and fluctuates, making the long-term effects of the MCP surgery and therapy difficult to define. Once more, large numbers of patients in each treatment group would be required to decrease the effects of attrition bias and to dilute the effects of subsequent interventions.

The difficulties of past studies guide the planning of future studies. Although the issues of low patient numbers, variable preoperative status, additional surgical and drug interventions, and chronic disease cannot be altered, study designs can. Large randomized trials may not be possible; however, samples of patients, paired according to preoperative status, may be allocated to different treatment protocols. Standardized measurement of pain, cosmesis, impairment, disability, and impact on the patient, made at similar postoperative time frames, would further assist in determining treatment efficacy.

5. Conclusion

This review suggests that *all* regimens contribute toward an increase in MCP motion and an increase in hand function, but despite the efforts of patients and clinicians, hand therapists remain unaware of the most effective postoperative protocol for MCP arthroplasty or the suitability of each regimen for specific implants and soft-tissue procedures. Difficulties in researching this topic include low patient numbers, highly variable preoperative status, lack of guidelines for outcome measures and time frames, and the effects of subsequent interventions received by the patient. The nature and size of the population with rheumatoid arthritis and MCP arthroplasty do not readily fit the randomized, controlled trial design. Paired sample designs are suggested, as well as the formation of standard outcome measures, for better comparison of results between patients.

6. References

[1] Krishnan J. The Biomechanical and Anatomical Basis for the Design of a New MCP Joint Prosthesis: [doctoral thesis], Australia: Flinders University School of Biomedical Engineering, 1998.

[2] Beevers DJ, Seedhom BB. Metacarpophalangeal joint prostheses. J Hand Surg. 1995;20B:125-36.

[3] Swanson AB. Silicone rubber implants for replacement of arthritic or destroyed joints in the hand. Surg Clin North Am. 1972;48:1113-27.

[4] Beiber EJ, Weiland AJ, Violenec-Dowling S. Silicone-rubber implant arthroplasty of the metacarpophalangeal joints for rheumatoid arthritis. J Bone Joint Surg [Am]. 1986;68:206-9.

[5] Pereira JA, Belcher HJCR. A comparison of metacarpophalangeal joint silastic arthroplasty with or without crossed intrinsic transfer. J Hand Surg. 2001;26B:229-34.

[6] Madden JW, De Vore G, Arem AJ. A rational post-operative program for metacarpophalangeal joint implant arthroplasty. J Hand Surg. 1977;2A:358-66.

[7] Clarke M, Oxman AD (eds). Cochrane Reviewers' Handbook 4.1.4. Oxford: The Cochrane Library, issue 4, update software, 2001.

[8] Ring D, Simmons BP, Hayes M. Continuous passive motion following metacarpophalangeal joint arthroplasty. J Hand Surg. 1998;23A:505–11.

[9] Thomsen NOB, Boeckstyns MEH and Leth-Espensen P. Value of dynamic splinting after replacement of the Metacarpophalangeal joint in patients with rheumatoid arthritis. Scand J Plast Reconstr Surg Hand Surg 2003; 37: 113–116.

[10] Groth G, Watkins M, Paynter P. Effect of an alternative flexion splinting protocol on mid-joint ROM [letter]. J Hand Ther. 1996;9:68-9.

[11] Burr N, Pratt AL, Smith PJ. An alternative splinting and rehabilitation protocol for metacarpophalangeal joint arthroplasty in patients with rheumatoid arthritis. J Hand Ther. 2002;15:41-7.

[12] Burr N, Pratt AL. MCP joint arthroplasty case study: the Mount Vernon static regime. Br J Hand Ther. 1999;4:137-40.

[13] Escott B, Ronald K and Judd M. NeuFlex and Swanson Metacarpophalangeal Implants for Rheumatoid Arthritis: Prospective Randomized, Controlled Clinical Trial Journal of Hand Surgery Volume 35, Issue 1, 2010, Pages 44-51.

[14] Harada Y, Okumura S and Takahashi Y. Hand Therapy After Metacarpophalangeal
     Joint Implant Arthroplasty in Rheumatoid Hand. Journal of Hand Therapy
     2010Volume 23, Issue 4, Pages e2-e3.
[15] Chung KC, Kotsis SV, and Kim HM, A Prospective Outcomes Study of Swanson
     Metacarpophalangeal Joint Arthroplasty for the Rheumatoid Hand. J Hand Surg
     Am. 2004 July; 29(4): 646–653.
Pettersson K, Wagnsjo P, Hulin E. NeuFlex compared with Sutterprostheses: a blind,
     prospective, randomized comparison of Silastic metacarpophalangeal joint
     prostheses. Scand J Plastic Reconstr Surg 2006;40:284 –290.
[16] V.A. Nuñez and N.D. Citron. Short-term results of the Ascension™ pyrolytic
     carbon metacarpophalangeal Joint replacement arthroplasty for osteoarthritis.
     Chirurgie de la Main. Volume 24, Issues 3-4, June-August 2005, Pages 161-
     164.
[17] Rettig LA, Luca L and Murphy MS. Silicone Implant Arthroplasty in Patients With
     Idiopathic Osteoarthritis of the Metacarpophalangeal Joint J Hand Surg
     2005;30A:667–672.
[18] Moller K, Sollerman C, Geijer M, Kopylov P, Ta¨gil M.Avanta versus Swanson silicone
     implants in the MCP joint -a prospective, randomized comparison of 30 patients
     followed for 2 years. J Hand Surg 2005;/30B:/8-13.
[19] Parkkila T , Belt EA, Markku Hakala M, Kautiainen H and Leppilahti J. Comparison of
     Swanson and Sutter Metacarpophalangeal Arthroplasties in Patients With
     Rheumatoid Arthritis: A Prospective and Randomized Trial Journal of Hand
     Surgery Volume 30, Issue 6, 2005, Pages 1276-1281
[20] Thomsen NOB, Michel E. H. Boeckstyns MEH and Leth-Espensen P. Value of
     dynamic splinting after replacement of the metacarpophalangeal joint in
     patients with rheumatoid arthritis. Scand J Plast Reconstr Surg Hand Surg
     2003; 37: 113–116
[21] Radmer S, Andresen S and Sparmann M. Poor experience with a hinged endoprosthesis
     (WEKO) for the metacarpophalangeal joints. Acta Orthop Scand 2003; 74 (5): 586–
     590.
[22] Ishikawa H, Murasawa A, Hanyu T (2002). The effects of activity andtype of
     rheumatoid   arthritis   on   the   flexible   implant   arthroplasty   ofthe
     metacarpophalangeal joint. Journal of Hand Surgery, 27B (2):180–183.
[23] Stothard J, Thompson AE and Sherris D. Correction of ulnar drift during silastic
     metacarpophalangeal joint arthroplasty. J Hand Surg (British Volume) 16B: 61-
     65.
[24] Sambandam SN Analysis of methodological deficiencies of studies reporting surgical
     outcome following cemented total-joint arthroplasty of trapezio-metacarpal joint of
     the thumb. Int Orthop 2007 31:639-45.
[25] Zhao C, Amadio PC, Zobitz ME, Momose T, Couvreur P, An K-N. Effect of synergistic
     motion on flexor digitorum profundus tendon excursion. Clin Orthop.
     2002;396:223-30.
[26] Tang JB, Wang B, Chen F, Chen Zhong Pan, Xie RG. Biomechanical evaluation of flexor
     tendon repair techniques. Clin Orthop. 2001;386:252-9.

[27] Tugwell P, Boers M. OMERACT conference on outcome measures in rheumatoid arthritis clinical trials: conclusion. J Rheumatol. 1993;20:590-1.

9

Development of Proprioception After Shoulder Arthroplasty

Michael W. Maier[1] and Philip Kasten[2]

[1]Department of Orthopedics, Trauma Surgery and Paraplegiology,
University of Heidelberg, Heidelberg
[2]Carl-Gustav Carus University of Dresden, Dresden
Germany

1. Introduction

Since the introduction of shoulder arthroplasty in 1893 by the French surgeon Jule-Émile Péan [18], the indications for shoulder replacement have expanded. Today shoulder arthroplasty is a common treatment for glenohumeral osteoarthritis [2]. Shoulder arthroplasty can significantly improve the function of osteoarthritic shoulders [7, 13, 19, 27]. Comparing the results, TSR offers better short- and mid-term results, but has the risk of long-term problems as the glenoid loosening [2]. In our practice patients with glenohumeral osteoarthritis will receive a total shoulder arthroplasty. As an exception patients with osteoarthritis which is limited to the humeral head without eccentric erosion of a stable sclerotic glenoid (Typ A1 glenoid according to Walch [28]) can be treated with hemiarthroplasty (HA). If the glenoid shows eccentric posterior wear (> A1), a TSR is recommended.

The use of total shoulder replacement in the setting of rotator cuff-tear arthropathy (CTA) has led to poor outcomes because of early glenoid implant failure [17]. These failures were the result of early glenoid loosening caused by altered biomechanics in the cuff-deficient shoulder. The treatment of choice for most used to be hemiarthroplasty. Although good relief from pain has usually been obtained, most patients with CTA and subsequent hemiarthroplasty had a limited range of movement, leading to difficulties with the activities of daily living. These poor results let to the development of the reverse shoulder prosthesis, as a new method for treating CTA. Using the reverse prosthesis in CTA, favorable outcomes have been reported [15, 17].

In order to use the replaced shoulder for ADLs the concerted function of the active stabilizers and the passive restraints of the replaced shoulder joint is necessary.

2. Shoulder proprioception

In 1906, Charles Scott Sherrington published his work about proprioception [26]. He defined the term proprioception as the awareness of movement derived from muscular, tendon, and articular sources. Since then physiologists and anatomists are searching for specialized nerve endings that transmit data on joint capsule and muscle tension [11, 30]. It is known that joint proprioception plays a considerable role in stabilization of the normal healthy shoulder by helping to control muscular action [1]. However, there is little data available about proprioception of the replaced shoulder before and after surgery [6, 12, 16]. Parameters routinely examined in previous studies include pain, satisfaction, range of motion, and strength [5].

3. Proprioception after shoulder arthroplasty

By reason that the shoulder joint is balanced and centered by the rotator cuff and the glenohumeral ligaments, it can be postulated that proprioception plays an important role in the postoperative outcome and rehabilitation. However, to date there are only three studies analyzing proprioception after shoulder replacement [6, 12, 16]. Two of these studies [6, 12] have a short follow-up period, in both cases six months. Cuomo et al. [6] performed a passive and guided angle-reproduction test in 20 patients with shoulder osteoarthritis before and six months after total shoulder arthroplasty (TSA) with only one degree of freedom at a time and reported improvement of proprioception [6]. Kasten et al. [12] found out, six months after shoulder arthroplasty, proprioception remained unchanged or deteriorated, as assessed by an active and unlimited angle-reproduction test with 3D motion analysis [12]. It was assumed that this finding was most likely attributable to the relatively short rehabilitation period of six months. Therefore, the purpose of the third study by Maier et al. [16] was to examine the patients from the study described by Kasten et al. [12, 14] again three years postoperatively to find out whether proprioception changes after a longer rehabilitation period of three years. In the present study, the same active and unlimited angle-reproduction test with 3D motion analysis was used as described before [12]. The present study firstly describes the results of proprioception development in a cohort of different shoulder arthroplasties, including patients with reverse prosthesis.

4. Measurement of proprioception

Because proprioception is a complex system that relies on central integration of various afferent and efferent elements, it is difficult to measure proprioceptive performance. Up to now, there is no consensus on how proprioception should be measured because the different components of proprioception are difficult to examine at the same time. For clinical purposes, most authors differentiate between static proprioception and dynamic proprioception [21]. Static proprioception is usually defined as the position sense, what means conscious perception of the orientation of different parts of the body with respect to another. Dynamic proprioception is defined as kinesthesia and the sense of rates of movement [11].

4.1 Joint angle analysis with the Heidelberg Upper Extremity Model (HUX)
In our studies [12, 16], we used the Heidelberg Upper Extremity Model (HUX) to measure joint angles as described before [23]: Therefore a twelve-camera motion analysis system (Vicon 612; Vicon, Lake Forest, USA) working at 120 Hz was used to monitor the patients' movements. The spatial resolution of the system was approximately 1 mm. The underlying model consisted of seven segments: thorax, clavicles, upper arms, and forearms. The sternoclavicular joint and the glenohumeral joint were treated as a ball-and-socket joint, whereas the elbow was treated as a hinge joint. Translational degrees of freedom were not considered in any of these joints.

For the measurement, the patients were prepared with four markers placed on the trunk as recommended by the International Society of Biomechanics [31]. Four markers were placed on each forearm: one at the radial and one at the ulnar styloid process of the wrist and two, connected with a wand, on the ulna close to the elbow joint. One marker was placed laterally on the upper arm and one on the acromion. After a static trial, the patient was asked to perform isolated movements of elbow flexion/ extension, shoulder flexion/ extension and shoulder abduction/ adduction to determine the shoulder joint position and the location of the elbow joint axis. Specifically, in these shoulder calibration trials the sternoclavicular joint was treated as a cardan joint. Technical coordinate systems for the ulna/ forearm, humerus, clavicle, and thorax were not deduced by optimization methods as was done for marker clusters [3]. Instead, they were based directly on marker trajectories, i.e. the direction vectors between them, using cross-products as reviewed by Chiari et al. [4]. The technical coordinate system of the clavicle was based on the four thorax markers and the shoulder marker. This coordinate system was used only for dynamic calibration movements, which were limited to a range of shoulder motion of 0-40° flexion and abduction to assume constant glenohumeral movement and exclude skin motion artefacts. Constraint least squares optimization according to Gamage et al. was then used for joint centre determination [9].

The anatomical co-ordinate system for the ulna/ forearm, humerus, and thorax were based on the technical coordinate systems of these segments and on the joint axes and joint centers previously determined. A static trial was used to define the neutral position of the thorax. Angles of flexion and abduction were expressed as projection angles relative to the proximal anatomical coordinate system, while internal/ external rotation was defined according to the globe convention [8]. Elbow flexion was defined as the projected angle to the elbow axis. Custom software written in Java (Sun Mircosystems, USA) was used to calculate each joint angle in each trial of the angle-reproduction tasks.

The system and biomechanical model was validated with the manual goniometer and intraclass correlation coefficients of 0.989 for intrasubject variability, 0.996 for intersubject variability, and 0.998 for intertester variability were found [22]. Differences of more than 10° between the two methods were found for shoulder flexion of more than 160° [22, 23].

4.2 Active angle reproduction test

As described before [12, 16], our study group used an active angle reproduction test to measure proprioception: Test person sat on a chair with the arm hanging in 0° abduction and rotation. They were blindfolded to eliminate visual clues and wore sleeveless shirts. We ensured that the arm did not touch the trunk and, consequently, skin contact was minimized. The arm was moved to the desired position by the examiner with visual control of a manual handheld goniometer. In detail, the positions were 30° and 60° abduction, 30° and 60° flexion, and 30° external (and afterwards 30° internal rotation) in 30° abduction (total six joint positions). In the target position the subjects were told to maintain the position for ten seconds, and then the initial position with the arm hanging was resumed. Afterwards, the subject was asked to move the arm back into the target position and the mean value of the joint position was measured. Standardized instructions were given to all subjects, and a test trial was conducted to acquaint them with each test condition. All tests were randomized for side and movement. Two test trials were performed at each angle, and the mean value was used for further analysis. The total proprioception performance (total) was defined as the mean value of all single measurements (six joint positions) to have one quality to compare proprioceptive ability.

5. Patients and controls

Patients receiving three different types of shoulder arthroplasties in 2007 were examined from 2007 to 2010:

i.   Ten consecutive patients underwent third-generation total shoulder arthroplasty (TSA) (Aequalis Shoulder; Tournier, Lyon, France) for degenerative osteoarthritis of the humeral head and glenoid with a mean age of 75 years (standard deviation [SD] 4.7 years). There were seven women and three men (mean height 167.0 cm [SD 11.0]; mean weight 81.0 kg [SD 15.9]), with four right shoulders and six left shoulders. In all cases the deltopectoral approach was used with detachment of the subscapularis tendon and release of all three glenohumeral ligaments. At the end of the surgery the subscapularis was reattached to the humeral bone. Primary osteoarthritis was found in eight cases and secondary posttraumatic osteoarthritis in two cases. The dominant side was involved in eight cases.

ii.   Eleven consecutive patients underwent hemiarthroplasty (HEMI) for degenerative changes limited to the humeral head and a stable/ minimally deformed glenoid of type A1 or A2 according to Walch [29]. There were nine women and two men, with five right shoulders and six left shoulders, four on the dominant sides and seven non-dominant sides. In all cases the deltopectoral approach was used as described above. Osteoarthritis was primary in nine cases and post-traumatic in two cases. The mean age was 64 years (SD 13.8), mean height was 167.0 cm (SD 8.1), and the mean weight was 79.0 kg (SD 18.8).

iii. In five patients a reversed prosthesis was implanted for cuff tear arthropathy (REVERSE). All were women, their mean age was 73 years (SD 4.6), mean height was 160 cm (SD 7.3), and mean weight was 73.6 kg (SD 7.4). In all cases the dominant right shoulder was treated. For all patients the anterior lateral approach was used with partial detachment of the anteriorlateral deltoid muscle and refixation in the end of the surgery. The subscapularis tendon and the glenohumeral ligaments at the glenoid were released.Consecutive patients were enrolled in the study which resulted in uneven numbers in the different groups of arthroplasties implanted. The main focus and outcome measure were not on comparing the groups (especially no comparison with the REVERSE group), but to monitor proprioception over time within the groups.

iv.   A matched control group consisted of five women and five men. Matched controls (n=10; NORM) had a mean age of 64.5 years (SD 7.3). The mean height was 170.3 cm (SD 9.3), and the mean weight was 78.2 kg (SD 11.6). All controls were right-hand dominant, healthy, and had normal shoulders according to medical history, physical examination and radiographs. In this group the test persons were also examined twice, over the period of three years.

6. Statistics

The statistical analysis was performed using SPSS Version 16.0 (SPSS Inc., Chicago, IL, USA). Group mean values (MV) and standard deviations (SD) were calculated. P values <0.05 were considered significant. The distribution of the data was checked with the

Shapiro-Wilk test, and the homogeneity of variance was assessed using the Levene test. The angle between the long axis of the humerus and the trunk position was determined. Differences in shoulder joint angles between target and reproducted position were compared between the pre- and postoperative examination with a Wilcoxon-test for the groups TSA, HEMI, and REVERSE. Afterwards as a second outcome measure differences among these groups and the controls were examined by a Mann-Whitney U test.

7. Results of proprioception measurement three years after shoulder arthroplasty

The hemioarthroplasty (HEMI) subgroup revealed significant lower AAR at 30° of external rotation before surgery with 3.1° [SD 3.5] as compared to three years after surgery 12.8° [SD 10.7]; (p=0.031) (fig. 1). By trend, in the TSA subgroup the AAR deteriorated from 7.1° [SD

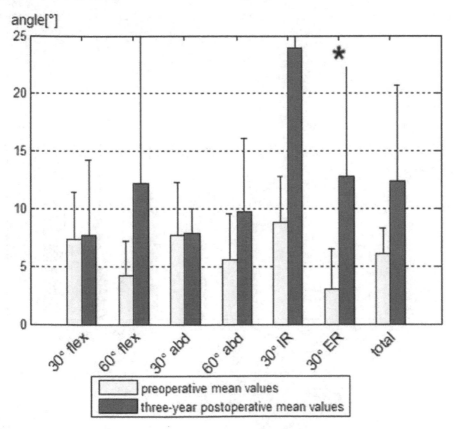

Fig. 1. The hemioarthroplasty (HEMI) group showed significant lower AAR at 30° of external rotation three years after surgery (3.1° [SD 3.5] vs. 12.8° [SD 10.7]; (p=0.031)). Otherwise there were no significances between pre- and postoperative AAR, although the total proprioception performance (total) almost reached significance (p=0.063). Graphically, there is a deterioration in all movements.

3.1] to 8.6° [SD 1.4] (fig. 2), in the HEMI subgroup from 6.1° [SD 2.1] to 12.4° [SD 8.3] (fig. 1) and in the reversed subgroup from 8.1° [SD 4.8] to 9.9° [SD 1.8] (fig. 3).

Although there are different underlying concepts and biomechanics between the TSA, HEMI and REVERSE group, the results were included in a combined analysis to get a general impression of the intervention of implantation of an arthroplasty: in all groups three years after shoulder arthroplasty the total proprioception performance (total) measured by the AAR deteriorated significantly (from 6.9° [SD 3.4] to 10.3° [SD 5.2]; p=0.018) (table 1). The internal rotation deteriorated significantly from 7.9° [SD 5.7] to 17.6° [SD 21.1] (p=0.039) (table 2). The comparison between the controls (NORM) and the three years postoperative values of all arthroplasty groups (TSA, HEMI and REVERSE) reveals a significant worse AAR in the arthroplasty group three years after shoulder arthroplasty (10.3° [SD 5.2] vs. 7.8° [SD 2.3]; p=0.030) (fig. 4).

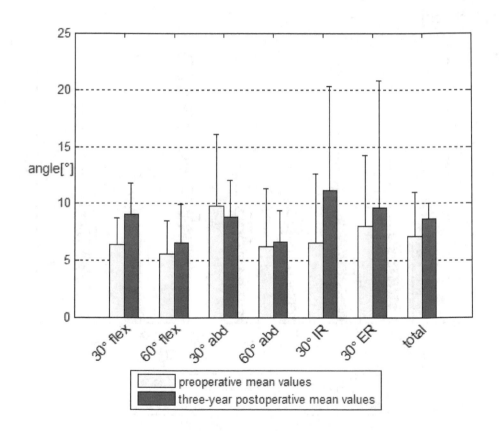

Fig. 2. The comparison pre- to postoperative values after implantation of a total shoulder arthroplasty (TSA) showed no significant differences between pre- and postoperative AAR. By trend, there is a deterioration of proprioception three years after surgery. The total proprioception performance (total) deteriorated by trend from 7.1° [SD 3.1] to 8.6° [SD 1.4].

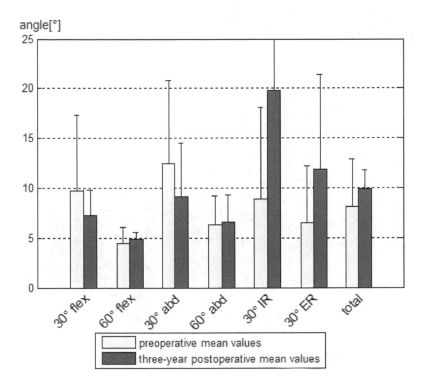

Fig. 3. The reversed shoulder arthroplasty (REVERSE) group graphically showed an improvement of the AAR at 30° of flexion and 30° of abduction. However, there is a deterioration for the other movements. The total proprioception performance (total) deteriorated by trend from 8.1° [SD 4.8] to 9.9° [SD 1.8].

Movement	Preoperatively		Three years postoperatively		P value
	Mean [°]	SD [°]	Mean [°]	SD [°]	
30° of flexion	7.4	± 4.1	8.2	± 4.3	0.669
60° of flexion	4.8	± 2.7	8.4	± 8.7	0.211
30° of abduction	9.5	± 5.7	8.5	± 3.1	0.562
60° of abduction	6.1	± 4.1	7.8	± 4.5	0.144
30° of external rotation	5.7	± 5.4	11.2	± 10.1	0.065
30° of internal rotation	7.9	± 5.7	17.6	± 21.1	**0.039**
Total	6.9	± 3.4	10.3	± 5.2	**0.018**

TSA total shoulder arthroplasty, *Hemi* hemiarthroplasty, *REVERSE* reversed arthroplasty, *SD* standard deviation;

Table 1. Active angle reproduction test (AAR) in all groups (TSA, HEMI and REVERSE) before operation and three years thereafter

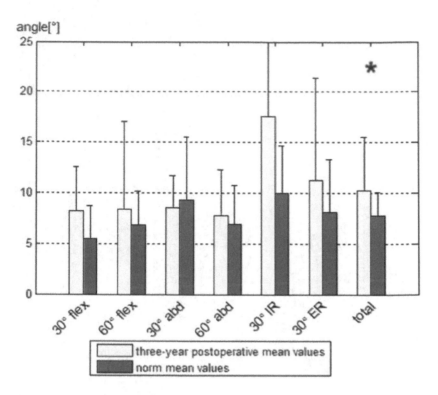

Fig. 4. The comparison between the controls and the three years postoperative values of all arthroplasty groups (TSA, HEMI and REVERSE) shows significantly better total proprioception performance (total) in the control (NORM) than in the arthroplasty group (10.3° [SD 5.2] vs. 7.8° [SD 2.3]; p=0.030).

8. Discussion of our findings with the literature

To our knowledge there are only three studies analyzing proprioception after shoulder arthroplasty [6, 12, 16]. Two are short-term studies with a six months follow-up [12, 16] and one is a middle-term follow up study [16]: Cuomo et al. [6] performed a prospective analysis of 20 consecutive patients with unilateral advanced glenohumeral arthritis who underwent total shoulder arthroplasty (TSA). Shoulder proprioception testing for passive position sense and detection of motion was performed one week before surgery and six months after TSA. Six months after TSA, position sense and the sensitivity of detection of motion were significantly improved (p<0.05) and did not differ significantly from the contralateral shoulder or the controls. Cuomo concluded that in patients with advanced glenohumeral arthritis after TSA there was a marked improvement in proprioception.

In our study group, Kasten et al. [12] assessed proprioception six months after shoulder arthroplasty by an *active* and unguided angle-reproduction test with 3D motion analysis. In contrast to Cuomo we found out that six months after surgery proprioception remained unchanged or deteriorated. Due to the fact that this is completely the different result as

Cuomo et. al., it was concluded, that this is either due to the different measurement methods (active versus passive) or the relatively short rehabilitation period of six months. Maybe an improvement would also be found in the mid-term follow-up. That's why we investigated the same patients three years after shoulder arthroplasty by the same active angle reproduction test to measure the development of proprioception [16]. The middl-term follow-up showed no improvement but rather a deterioration of proprioception over the course of three years after shoulder arthroplasty. How can we explain that?

Cuomo et al. used a hydraulic machine that passively moved the arm. The patient had to indicate when he or she noted movement ("detection of motion") and, in a separate approach, when he or she passively reassumed a joint position that was previously defined ("passive position sense"). Cuomo and colleagues thus measured two entities of proprioception separately. The outcome of the AAR test, used in our setting, can be influenced by some elements: The test person has to actively move the arm and is therefore not limited regarding the direction of movement. Consequently, a more comprehensive concept of proprioception is tested, comprising the elements of position sense, motion sense, and the muscle strength that is necessary to reassume the position.

9. Proprioception in shoulder instability

The AAR has been used to assess shoulder proprioception before, for example, in shoulder instability. Pötzl and colleagues examined the proprioceptive capabilities of 14 patients with recurrent anterior shoulder instability preoperatively and at least five years postoperatively using the AAR test [20]. In their series the joint position sense improved significantly in abduction, flexion, and rotation (p<0.05). They concluded that five years after surgical restoration of shoulder instability the joint position sense improved significantly to the same level as normal healthy shoulders. Having these results in mind we have to ask why proprioception measured with a comparable AAR deteriorates after shoulder arthroplasty, whereas it improves after surgery of shoulder instability?

10. Possible reasons why proprioception deteriorates after shoulder arthroplasty

In shoulder arthroplasty, the operative approach for implantation of a TSA and hemi-arthroplasty includes the cutting (and subsequent repair) of the subscapularis muscle and usually release of all glenohumeral ligaments. In cuff tear arthropathy the subscapularis is damaged from the beginning or released during surgery in our technique. However, these structures contain afferent and efferent structures important for proprioception. Therefore, concerning the influence on proprioceptive structures, the surgical procedures for shoulder instability and shoulder replacement are distinct. Since the approach in TSA and hemiarthroplasty is identical, a comparison seems to be valid. The different approach and the lack of the rotator cuff in cuff tear arthropathy limits a direct comparison with the other groups. However, the aim of this study was not the comparison of different types of implants that were implanted for different indications. The aim of this study was to assess proprioception changes three years after shoulder arthroplasty within the three groups. What we observed in our study is that nociceptors may also play an important role. During the repeat postoperative measurement, the patients mentioned that they were lacking the information input of pain sensation that they had usually during motion of the arm before surgery. The lacking of this afferent input might adversely influence the postoperative proprioception performance with the AAR.

11. What can we do to avoid postoperative deterioration of proprioception?

Another issue is how we could diminish the loss of proprioception after shoulder replacement. Certainly we have to take a look at the surgical procedure. In the cases of TSA and HEP the deltopectoral approach was used with detachment of the subscapularis tendon and release of all glenohumeral ligaments. In shoulder replacement different procedures exist for detachment of the subscapularis tendon. If the external rotation is > 20°, according to our concept the subscapularis tendon is divided 5-10 mm medial to its insertion at the lesser tuberosity. The lateral tendon stump will permit an end-to-end suture at the end of surgery. If the external rotation is <20°, the detachment of the subscapularis tendon from the lesser tuberosity is recommended, because this allows to gain length by medializing the tendon insertion after implantation of the prosthesis. At the end of the surgery, the subscapularis tendon is repaired in slight abduction and external rotation of the arm either with an end-to-end suture or, in the presence of joint contracture, reattached with the help of previously mounted transosseous sutures [10, 24]. This refixation is important, because otherwise it carries the risk of a later anterior instability of the prosthesis and loss of shoulder function.

This intraoperative soft tissue management could play an important role for the proprioceptive outcome according to a recently published study by Rokito et al. [25]. They investigated the degree to which surgical approach affects recovery of strength and proprioception. The recovery of strength and proprioception after open surgery for recurrent anterior glenohumeral instability was compared for two surgical procedures. Group 1 underwent an open inferior capsular shift with detachment of the subscapularis, and group 2 underwent an anterior capsulolabral reconstruction without detachment of the subscapularis. In group 1 the subscapularis was split horizontally at the junction of its upper two-third and lower one-third, and a glenoid-sided capsular shift was performed, followed by reapproximation of the split. At 6 months after surgery in group 1 patients there were still significant deficits in mean position sense and strength values. Rokito concluded that detachment of the subscapularis delays recovery of strength and proprioception. These findings can explain the deterioration of proprioceptive outcome in shoulder arthroplasty which usually implies the detachment of the subscapularis muscle. Another important issue is the release of the glenohumeral ligaments that play an important role in proprioception of the shoulder. Postoperative management with immobilizing in a Gilchrist sling or an abduction pillow, physiotherapy management including a temporary avoidance for rotational movements to allow for healing of the subscapularis muscle as well as proprioceptive neuromuscular facilitation exercises might play an important role for the individual proprioceptive outcome.

Performing shoulder arthroplasty did negatively affect one component of shoulder proprioception that was measured by the active angle-reproduction test. This might be related to the surgical approach that includes divison of the subscapularis muscle and the glenohumeral ligaments. In order to be able to diminish negative influences on postoperative proprioception further prospective studies will have to evaluate pre- and intraoperative variables to improve proprioception after shoulder replacement. Although proprioception does not improve three years after implantation of shoulder arthroplasty, a pain free increase of range of motion in activities of daily living, as we described in a previous study [13], is the main improvement for the patient after surgery.

Summary sentence

Shoulder proprioception deteriorates after shoulder arthroplasty.

Disclosures

All authors, their immediate family, and any research foundation with which they are affiliated did not receive any financial payments or other benefits from any commercial entity related to the subject of this article.

Source of funding

Research fund of the Department of Orthopaedic and Trauma Surgery of the Hospital of the University of Heidelberg.
The local ethics committee approved the study (S-305/2007) and all patients consented to the study.

12. Aknowledgements

We thank the research fund of the Department of Orthopaedic and Trauma Surgery of the Hospital of the University of Heidelberg for the financial support of the study. Furthermore, we would like to thank the motion analysis team of the University of Heidelberg, especially Petra Armbrust and Waltraud Schuster, for the practical support during the study.[Level of Evidence : Level III, Case-Control Study, Treatment Study.

13. References

[1] Blasier, R.B., J.E. Carpenter, and L.J. Huston, Shoulder proprioception. Effect of joint laxity, joint position, and direction of motion. Orthop.Rev., 1994. 23(1): p. 45-50.
[2] Boileau, P., et al., Arthroplasty of the shoulder. J.Bone Joint Surg.Br., 2006. 88(5): p. 562-575.
[3] Carman, A.B. and P.D. Milburn, Determining rigid body transformation parameters from ill-conditioned spatial marker co-ordinates. J Biomech, 2006. 39(10): p. 1778-86.
[4] Chiari, L., et al., Human movement analysis using stereophotogrammetry. Part 2: instrumental errors. Gait Posture, 2005. 21(2): p. 197-211.
[5] Constant, C.R. and A.H. Murley, A clinical method of functional assessment of the shoulder. Clin Orthop Relat Res., 1987(214): p. 160-164.
[6] Cuomo, F., M.G. Birdzell, and J.D. Zuckerman, The effect of degenerative arthritis and prosthetic arthroplasty on shoulder proprioception. J Shoulder Elbow Surg, 2005. 14(4): p. 345-348.
[7] Deshmukh, A.V., et al., Total shoulder arthroplasty: long-term survivorship, functional outcome, and quality of life. J Shoulder Elbow Surg, 2005. 14(5): p. 471-9.
[8] Doorenbosch, C.A., J. Harlaar, and D.H. Veeger, The globe system: an unambiguous description of shoulder positions in daily life movements. J Rehabil Res Dev, 2003. 40(2): p. 147-55.
[9] Gamage, S.S. and J. Lasenby, New least squares solutions for estimating the average centre of rotation and the axis of rotation. J Biomech, 2002. 35(1): p. 87-93.

[10] Habermeyer, P. and G. Engel, *Surgical technique for total shoulder arthroplasty.* Operat Orthop Traumatol, 2004. 16: p. 339-364.

[11] Jerosch, J. and M. Prymka, *Proprioception and joint stability.* Knee.Surg.Sports Traumatol.Arthrosc., 1996. 4(3): p. 171-179.

[12] Kasten, P., et al., *Proprioception in total, hemi- and reverse shoulder arthroplasty in 3D motion analyses: a prospective study.* Int Orthop, 2009. 33(6): p. 1641-7.

[13] Kasten, P., et al., *Can shoulder arthroplasty restore the range of motion in activities of daily living? A prospective 3D video motion analysis study.* J Shoulder Elbow Surg, 2010. 19(2 Suppl): p. 59-65.

[14] Kasten, P., et al., *Three-dimensional motion analysis of compensatory movements in patients with radioulnar synostosis performing activities of daily living.* J Orthop Sci, 2009. 14(3): p. 307-12.

[15] Loew, M., et al., *[Shoulder arthroplasty following rotator cuff tear: acquired arthropathy of the shoulder].* Orthopade, 2007. 36(11): p. 988-95.

[16] Maier, M.W., et al., *Proprioception three years after shoulder arthroplasty in 3D motion analysis: a prospective study.* submitted to Int Orthop, 2011.

[17] Matsen, F.A., 3rd, et al., *The reverse total shoulder arthroplasty.* J Bone Joint Surg Am, 2007. 89(3): p. 660-7.

[18] Nyffeler, R.W., et al., *Influence of humeral prosthesis height on biomechanics of glenohumeral abduction. An in vitro study.* J Bone Joint Surg Am, 2004. 86-A(3): p. 575-80.

[19] Orfaly, R.M., et al., *A prospective functional outcome study of shoulder arthroplasty for osteoarthritis with an intact rotator cuff.* J Shoulder Elbow Surg, 2003. 12(3): p. 214-21.

[20] Potzl, W., et al., *Proprioception of the shoulder joint after surgical repair for Instability: a long-term follow-up study.* Am.J.Sports Med., 2004. 32(2): p. 425-430.

[21] Proske, U. and S.C. Gandevia, *The kinaesthetic senses.* J Physiol, 2009. 587(Pt 17): p. 4139-46.

[22] Raiss, P., et al., *[Range of motion of shoulder and elbow in activities of daily life in 3D motion analysis].* Z.Orthop.Unfall., 2007. 145(4): p. 493-498.

[23] Rettig, O., et al., *A new kinematic model of the upper extremity based on functional joint parameter determination for shoulder and elbow.* Gait Posture, 2009. 30(4): p. 469-76.

[24] Rockwood, C.A., Jr., *The technique of total shoulder arthroplasty.* Instr Course Lect, 1990. 39: p. 437-47.

[25] Rokito, A.S., et al., *Recovery of shoulder strength and proprioception after open surgery for recurrent anterior instability: a comparison of two surgical techniques.* J Shoulder Elbow Surg, 2010. 19(4): p. 564-9.

[26] Sherrington, C.S., *On the proprioceptive system, especially in its reflex aspect.* Brain, 1906. 29: p. 1-28.

[27] van de Sande, M.A., R. Brand, and P.M. Rozing, *Indications, complications, and results of shoulder arthroplasty.* Scand J Rheumatol, 2006. 35(6): p. 426-34.

[28] Walch, G., P. Boileau, and P. Pozzi, *Glenoid resurfacing in shoulder arthroplasty.* In: Walch G, Boileau P, eds.: Shoulder arthroplasty.Berlin, Heidelberg, New York, Tokio: Springer, 1999: p. 177-181.

[29] Walch, G., et al., *Primary glenohumeral osteoarthritis: clinical and radiographic classification. The Aequalis Group.* Acta Orthop.Belg., 1998. 64 Suppl 2: p. 46-52.

[30] Warner, J.J., et al., *Static capsuloligamentous restraints to superior-inferior translation of the glenohumeral joint.* Am.J.Sports Med., 1992. 20(6): p. 675-685.

[31] Wu, G., et al., *ISB recommendation on definitions of joint coordinate systems of various joints for the reporting of human joint motion--Part II: shoulder, elbow, wrist and hand.* J Biomech, 2005. 38(5): p. 981-992.

10

Humeral Hemiarthroplasty with Spherical Glenoid Reaming: Theory and Technique of The Ream and Run Procedure

Moby Parsons
Seacoast Orthopedics and Sports Medicine
Somersworth, NH
USA

1. Introduction

Despite improvements in glenoid prosthesis design, materials and surgical techniques, complications related to the glenoid component continue to be a leading cause of failure after total shoulder arthroplasty. Although previously felt to be of little clinical significance, radiolucent lines around the glenoid prosthesis are now recognized as a sign of impending mid and long term fixation problems. While much attention in shoulder prosthesis design has focused on anatomical reconstruction of the humerus through increasing modularity, comparatively little progress has been made in solving the problems of glenoid wear and fixation failure. Resolving these issues on the socket side of the equation remains a challenge for the shoulder arthroplasty surgeon as the population ages, as young patients present with terminal shoulder arthritis and as patients demand higher performance from their implant.

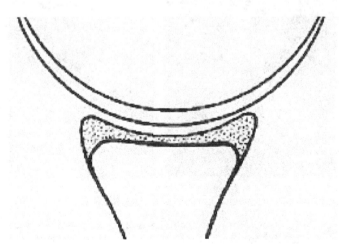

Fig. 1. In the normal glenohumeral joint, the compliance of the articular cartilage and the labrum provide for conforming surfaces which optimize stability and load distribution.

In the normal shoulder, the compliance of the articular cartilage and labrum allow the mating surfaces to conform under applied loads throughout a wide range of motion (Figure 1). Thus, normal, physiological glenohumeral translations can occur between congruent surfaces without introducing a kinematic conflict caused by excessive constraint. Because polyethylene glenoids are not compliant, they cannot instantly deform to remain congruent as normal translations occur. To resolve the potential conflict between conformity and constraint, total shoulder systems have introduced mismatch between the radii of curvature of the head and glenoid to permit small translations that increase range of motion and resolve some of the stresses transmitted to the fixation interface.

While mismatch has proven to reduce earlier fixation failure, it also facilitates eccentric loading by allowing the center of rotation of the humerus to translate away form the center of the glenoid concavity. As the contact point on the prosthetic glenoid surface changes, there are corresponding marked changes in the cement mantle stress than ultimately result in micromotion at the bone cement interface.[1] Oosterom and colleagues performed biomechanical studies looking at the effect of varying degrees of conformity on rim loading and found that mismatch increases rim displacement.[2] Furthermore, mismatch results in abrasive wear at the prosthetic surface and a higher likelihood of material failure under eccentric loading conditions.[3] Retrieval studies of failed glenoids that have radial mismatch, have repeatedly shown characteristic changes in the prosthetic surface including edge deformation, rim fracture, broad surface irregularity and wear to conformity (Figure 2).[4,5]

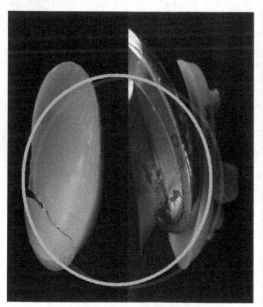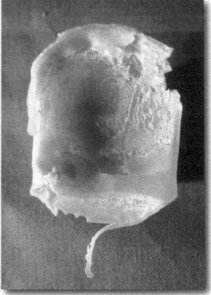

Fig. 2. Wear to conformity (left), broad surface abrasion and rim wear (right).

Modes of damage have been found most commonly in the inferior quadrant suggesting calcar impingement with the humerus.[6] Braman et al further showed that alterations in the surface geometry of the damaged prosthesis compromised its intrinsic stability, thus exacerbating the pathomechanics that result in surface damage to begin with.[4]

Several studies have looked at glenoid prosthesis design parameters and at cementation and bone preparation techniques seeking to optimize fixation to the host bone and resist tensile stresses imparted by eccentric loading conditions.[8-10] There is general consensus that pegged glenoid components tend to outperform keeled components and that third generation cementation techniques have reduced the incidence of early radiolucent lines. While most outcome studies show survivorship of the prosthesis at midterm, clinical outcome studies demonstrate deterioration in glenoid component longevity as the time interval from surgery increases. Walch and colleagues in a multicenter study of 333 shoulder arthroplasties performed with the same cemented convex-backed glenoid component showed that nearly 50% were radiographically loose at 10 years.[11] The need to eccentrically ream the glenoid to correct posterior erosion was associated with a higher rate of loosening. Young et al performed a similar multicenter study looking at long-term survivorship of a cemented flat-backed, keeled all-polyethylene glenoids and found radiographic loosening of 20% at 10 years and 67% at 15 years.[12] Kasten et al similarly noted at 9% rate of loosening at 5 years, which increased to 33% at 9 years. Radiolucent lines were noted to progress over time.[13] As with arthroplasty of other joints that rely on cement fixation, progressive radiolucency is an "at risk" sign for eventual loosening and though mid-term data show little correlation between lucency and revision, it is expected that longer follow-up will bear out eventual clinical failure. Bartelt et al followed a cohort of patients younger than age 55 years who underwent total shoulder arthroplasty and found a 30% rate of radiographic loosening at a mean of 6.6 years.[14] The implant survival rate in this group was only 92% at 10 years.

In light of these sobering data, there have been historical and resurging attempts to improve fixation durability by capitalizing on the proven success of bone ingrowth into porous metal surfaces. However, experience with early metal-backed designs demonstrated failure rates much higher than for cemented polyethylene components.[15] Taunton et al reported on revision or radiographic failure for a metal-backed, bone-growth glenoid of 20% at 5 years and 48% at 10 years.[16] Unacceptably high rates of radiographic failure have also been reported for cemented metal-backed glenoid components.[17] Although some cases of fibrous ingrowth have been documented, many of these failures were not related to fixation problems between the metal and the bone, rather to excessive polyethylene wear, locking mechanism problems and severe osteolysis.[18] Tensile stress seems to be transferred to the fixation between the polyethylene and metal baseplates leading to the potential for excessive wear, fracture and dissociation of the components. While much of this experience is based on implants used in the 1980's to 1990's, there is renewed interest in metal-backed designs given the success of metal base plates in reverse shoulder arthroplasty and the desire to have modularity on the glenoid side facilitating conversion between primary and reverse shoulder replacement. Clinical outcome studies on newer designs have yet to prove their merit versus their historical counterparts and the current standard set by cemented all polyethylene designs, albeit a fair standard compared to survivorship data for hip and knee arthroplasty.

These data are alarming considering the growing epidemic of degenerative conditions in younger patients, the higher expectations of patients who wish to remain physically active into their older years and the general aging of the population. The conclusion one can draw from the current clinical and basic science literature is that modern prosthetic glenoid components are destined to fail by wear and loosening with repeated eccentric loading. Thus, for younger patients or those whose life-expectancy is greater than 15 years there is a high likelihood that revision surgery will be necessary to address glenoid component failure. In many of these cases, reimplantation of a glenoid component is not possible due to structural deficiency of the remaining glenoid vault, and functional outcomes are often uncertain.[19,20] Studies on structural grafting of bone deficits have shown a high rate of short-term reconstitution but long-term subsidence indicating that durable and reliable solutions for the failed glenoid are not yet available for this growing cohort of patients.[21,22]

To address the need for surgical options to treat shoulder arthritis in younger patients, biological resurfacing procedures using a number of different interposition materials have been evaluated with largely varying short and mid-term success. Autogenous fascia lata, Achilles tendon[23-24] and glenohumeral capsule,[25,26] allograft lateral meniscus[27,28] and dermal scaffolds,[29] and xenographic tissues patches[30] have all been used to resurface the worn glenoid. Both arthroscopic and open techniques have been reported and techniques have included humeral chondroplasty, humeral prosthetic surface replacement versus stemmed humeral hemiarthroplasty.[23] While some of these reports demonstrate initial improvement in pain and function, progressive joint space narrowing and glenoid erosion are common and consequent eventual revision to definitive arthroplasty. Gerber has nicely summarized the literature on this field, stating "Biologic resurfacing of the glenoid has hitherto failed to adequately restore the geometry and biology of the glenoid."[31] It is fair to say that lesser invasive approaches such as the arthroscopic techniques can be used as an interval step to delay arthroplasty but durable long-term results from these procedures seem to be the exception rather than the rule.

Hemiarthroplasty without glenoid resurfacing or reshaping is yet another alternative to total shoulder replacement which avoids the risk of glenoid failure. There has been extensive comparison between hemiarthroplasty and total shoulder arthroplasty in the literature looking at comparative outcomes. It is fairly well-established based on these studies including a meta-analysis of the existing literature, that total shoulder arthroplasty provides superior pain relief and range of motion over time.[32-34] Nevertheless, some series do show comparable outcomes recognizing that some patients with progressive glenoid erosion do require conversion to total shoulder arthroplasty.[35] Levine et al have shown that results of hemiarthroplasty are inferior if preoperative glenoid erosion or posterior wear exists.[36] This highlights the importance of recentering the humeral head and restoring proper load-bearing mechanics at the glenohumeral joint after prosthetic reconstruction. Sperling and colleagues studied long-term results of hemiarthroplasty versus total shoulder in patients 50 years or younger.[33] While glenoid wear after hemiarthroplasty was present in 72% of cases, radiolucencies around the glenoid prosthesis were present in 76% of patients. The risk of painful glenoid erosion necessitating revision glenoid replacement lead to the conclusion that patients with total shoulder replacement have superior clinical outcomes. The authors also concluded however based on survivorship of total shoulders in this cohort that "great care must be exercised, and alternative methods of treatment considered before either hemiarthroplasty or total shoulder arthroplasty is offered to patients aged 50 years or younger."

Based on this background, a definitive treatment option for young and physically demanding patients with end-stage shoulder arthritis remains both a need and a challenge. Experience with the failure modes of both hemiarthroplasty and total shoulder arthroplasty, along with a better understanding of glenohumeral biomechanics have laid a foundation on which such a treatment must be based to provided a lasting solution that withstands the rigors in which many of these patients wish to engage. In 1992, Frederick A. Matsen, III, MD began investigating the technique of humeral hemiarthroplasty with spherical glenoid reaming to restore a concavity to the glenoid and to reorient the worn glenoid perpendicular to the centerline of the scapular body. This technique has hence become known as the Ream and Run procedure. As follows is an in-depth description of basic science and clinical support for this technique, the principles of its application, patient selection, surgical technique, recovery and results.

2. Basic science and clinical support

According to Matsen, "glenoid components fail as a result of their inability to replicate essential properties of the normal glenoid articular surface to achieve durable fixation to the underlying bone, to withstand repeated eccentric loads and glenohumeral translation, and to resist wear and deformation."[37] The Ream and Run seeks to address these deficiencies by stimulating a biological response at the glenoid surface that can adapt to the applied stress through the process of healing and remodeling. Interest in this potential came from observations on retrieval studies of mold arthroplasty of the hip. Observations on this historical technique showed that the reamed acetabular bone was often covered with a smooth fibrous tissue layer that amounted to a biological resurfacing.[38] In addition, histologic studies demonstrated a relatively normal subchondral bony architecture that had remodeled according to the loads born on the surface.[39, 40] Failure of this technique was often due to loosening and bone resorption on the femoral side.[41] These results suggest that reamed bone has a regenerative potential to yield a durable joint surface when articulating with a convex metallic prosthesis.

Laboratory studies were then undertaken to determine if the reamed glenoid concavity was comparatively stable to either the native or a prosthetic glenoid. Weldon et al, using a cadaveric model, demonstrated that the intrinsic glenoid stability was compromised by loss of articular cartilage and that this stability could be restored to levels comparable to a prosthetic glenoid through spherical reaming.[42] In other words, the surface geometry of the bone predicts its influence on glenohumeral kinematics. To further characterize the healing process that occurs at the reamed glenoid surface, Matsen and colleagues performed histologic analysis of retrieved glenoids at serial follow-up intervals in a canine model of the Ream and Run.[43] At 24 weeks post-surgery specimens consistently showed growth of a thick fibrocartilaginous tissue covering and firmly attached to the glenoid surface.(Figure 3) This progressive maturation between 3 and 6 months and remained congruent with the articulating humeral hemiarthroplasty.

The implication of these findings are: 1) healing and remodeling of the reamed bone is a progressive process demonstrating continued biological activity in response to the mechanical environment; and 2) progressive maturation of the regenerative surface suggests its ability to withstand its mechanical environment.

Based on this background, the Ream and Run procedure been in clinical application now for well over a decade, and its indications and techniques have been refined with increasing experience. As the length of follow-up continues for these patients, the foundations for sustained positive outcomes and the modes of failure have become clearer. These foundations are anchored in the principles behind this technique all of which relate to replicating the anatomical relationships of the glenohumeral joint and the biomechanical properties these relationships engender.

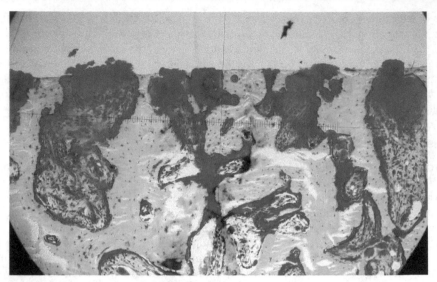

Fig. 3. Fibrocartilage growth between reamed boney trabeculae.

3. Principles

The key principles behind the Ream and Run which the surgeon must consider in reestablishing a lasting articulation that can withstand wear can be remembered as the 4 Cs: concavity, conformity, centerline and center of rotation. These are further discussed as follows.

3.1 Concavity

Stability of the glenohumeral joint in the midrange relies on dynamic centering of the humeral head into the glenoid concavity by the force couples generated by the rotator cuff. Coordination between the rotator cuff and periscapular stabilizing muscles ensures that the net reaction force at the glenohumeral joint is directed within the confines of the glenoid concavity. The depth and shape of this concavity can affect stability by altering the glenoids ability to contain the resultant force from shoulder motion. This can be measured as the balance stability angle (BSA) – the maximal angle the net humeral reaction force vector can make with the glenoid centerline before the head dislocates.[42] Both the width and the depth of the glenoid factor into the intrinsic stability and these, in turn, can be affected both by pathologic changes from arthritis as well as by corrective reaming.

Reestablishing a smooth concavity with sufficient depth and surface area is a central goal of the successful Ream and Run. Because reaming affects both depth and width, depending on the degree of necessary correction to recenter the humeral head, careful attention must be paid through preoperative planning and precise surgical technique to restore a sufficient concavity without compromising other principles as will be subsequently discussed. In cases where there is severe posterior glenoid wear, as can occur from capsulorraphy arthropathy, corrective reaming to restore glenoid version may sacrifice too much surface area in order to restore a sufficient concavity thus obviating the benefit of this procedure. Prosthetic glenoid resurfacing may be necessary in such cases despite the inherent risks of eventual failure.

3.2 Conformity

Although the boney anatomy is not conforming between the humeral head and glenoid concavity, the compliance afforded by the articular cartilage and glenoid labrum provide for conformity and congruency as the humeral head is centered and compressed. It is this conformity and compliance that permits load distribution over the glenoid face. Because bone and polyethylene are not as compliant as cartilage and labrum, some degree of mismatch between the diameter of curvature of the humeral head and glenoid has become a convention in total shoulder arthroplasty to avoid excessive constraint and allow physiologic translations. While historically mismatch seems to improve the longevity of prosthetic glenoid fixation, translations also allow eccentric glenoid loading, which contributes to eventual fixation failure. Mismatch also affects load distribution by concentrating loads over a smaller surface area on the glenoid surface.

In principle, the Ream and Run procedure must respect the biomechanical principles on which glenohumeral stability and load transfer are based while simultaneously reconciling the kinematic conflict that occurs between conformity and constraint as is seen with prosthetic glenoids. Stability is afforded by creation of a concavity into which the head can be centered after appropriate releases have been performed. Preservation of the labrum further deepens the socket and improves congruency between the ball and socket. Load distribution is optimized by choosing a mismatch of 2mm, which reduces point contact but allows some forgiveness in terms of constraint. It also provides some forgiveness in allowing the prosthetic humeral head to chose a centering point about which adaptive remodeling of the glenoid surface can define the final shape that optimizes joint kinematics and load transfer.

3.3 Centerline

In the normal shoulder, the glenoid is retroverted on average 10 degrees. The glenoid centerline (the line perpendicular to the glenoid face) thus normally points 10 degrees posterior to the axis of the scapular body. This line exits the scapula anteriorly at the base of the glenoid vault between the superior and inferior subscapularis crurae. Recentering the humeral head within the glenoid concavity is essential for shoulder mobility, stability and load transfer. The pathomechanics of primary and secondary arthritis often lead to posterior subluxation of the humerus and consequent posterior glenoid wear and erosion. These pathologic changes must be corrected to optimize load-bearing mechanics at the joint after prosthetic reconstruction. As will be discussed later, careful planning is necessary to determine the amount of correction that will restore the orientation of the glenoid.(Figure 4) Reorientation of the glenoid concavity through corrective reaming can diminish the surface area of the articulation because the glenoid vault narrows as one moves medially. In addition, corrective reaming to "bring down the high side" may result in significant penetration of the subchondral bone, which is softer and less tolerant of bearing significant loads when articulating with a convex metal prosthesis. Medialization of the glenoid may also increase the reaction force at the glenohumeral joint by reducing the lever arm of the rotator cuff muscles and may result in secondary impingement by bringing the tuberosity underneath the lateral acromion. Thus, preoperative planning must assess the degree of necessary correction and whether this will exceed the anatomical parameters necessary to achieve the other principles and goals of the Ream and Run.

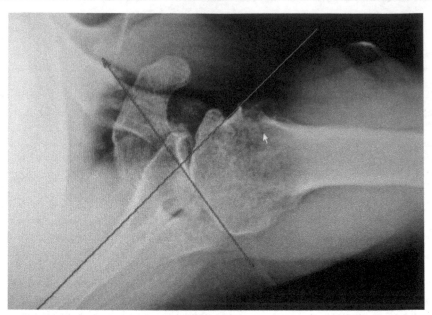

Fig. 4. Axillary lateral radiograph showing double concavity, posterior glenoid erosion and posterior humeral subluxation. Preoperative planning can determine the degree of corrective reaming needed to restore proper glenoid orientation relative to the axis of the scapula

In cases where significant correction is required, precontouring the glenoid with a burr and then using a relatively flatter conventional reamer to start may allow reorientation without as much medialization and subchondral penetration. Some surgeons have advocated under correction of the posterior erosion to maximize the articular surface area of the reamed glenoid.[44] While undercorrection risks recurrent posterior instability and consequent wear, excessive reaming risks reduced surface area for load distribution. Ultimately, the surgeon needs to make a judgment call intraoperatively after corrective reaming as to whether the concavity can sufficiently replicate the mechanical properties of a normal glenoid to provide lasting pain relief, stability and unrestricted function.

3.4 Center of rotation
Because the humeral head is nearly spherical, it has a center of rotation, which is slightly medially and posteriorly offset from the axis of the humeral shaft. In the normal shoulder this rotation center is aligned with center of the glenoid concavity. This phenomenon has been termed glenohumeral register.[44] This center of rotation actually exists within a larger arc of a sphere created by the coracoacromial arch and coracoid process – a boundary which partially constrains glenohumeral motion and helps define the path of rotation.(Figure 5) The motion of the humeral articular surface on the glenoid face can actually be described as slippage of the surfaces relative to one another. The centering point on the glenoid can thus be thought of as a slippage point. In the normal shoulder, this point is slightly inferior and anterior to the midpoint of Saller's line which bisects the glenoid along its superior to inferior axis.

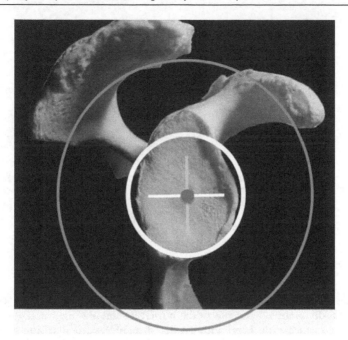

Fig. 5. The centering point on the glenoid is defined by the larger sphere created by the coracoacromial arch. The point is slightly inferior to the center of a line connecting the superior and inferior margins of the glenoid.

Anatomical reconstruction of the proximal humerus seeks to reestablish the head to tuberosity and head to shaft relationships and to replace a head of similar diameter and thickness. In a perfect world, this should restore the proper center of rotation though prior studies have shown that there can be significant displacement of the rotation center depending on how the chosen system fits relative to a given patient's anatomy. [45, 46] (Figure 6) This displacement has the potential to affect the location of the slippage point on the glenoid face and how the motion of the glenohumeral joint is defined by its location with fornix humeri.

When the glenoid is spherically reamed, the surgeon is effectively choosing a centering point for slippage of the humeral prosthesis. Much of the time in conventional shoulder arthroplasty, this point is chosen by looking at what appears to be the deepest point of the existing concavity. Current techniques and technology do not allow the reconstructed center of rotation of the humerus to chose it's proper slippage point that the surgeon can then use as the centering point for the reaming. The finding on failed glenoid retrievals that wear to conformity occurs at a point other than the geometric center of the prosthetic glenoid concavity, suggests that the humeral head is seeking ball and socket kinematics as defined by placement of the reconstructed humeral rotation center within the fornix humeri. Thus, one can presume that optimal registration between the rotation center of the humeral arthroplasty and the center of the reamed glenoid concavity would result in a blend of kinematics, stability and load distribution that would lend itself to long-term maintenance of pain relief and function.

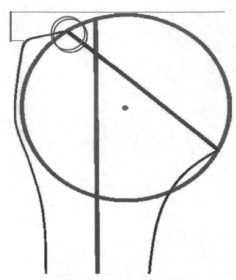

Fig. 6. Anatomical prosthetic reconstruction of the proximal humerus should seeks to restore the center of rotation relative to the axis of the humeral shaft and the transition between the superior articular surface of the head with the insertion of the articular side of the rotator cuff on the greater tuberosity

In the absence of a scientific method to register the humeral reconstruction with the slippage point on the reamed glenoid, the shoulder arthroplasty surgeon must resort to preoperative planning, intraoperative observation, precise surgical technique and perhaps a bit of good fortune. While the reamed glenoid bone is not as compliant as articular cartilage, it does have the capacity to adapt and remodel according to its mechanical environment and thus, over time there may be some forgiveness to a small margin of error through a process of bedding-in wear.

4. Indications

Proper patient selection is critical to achieving desired results after this procedure. Selection is based both on anatomical and physiological considerations as well emotional and social aspects of the patient. Foremost, patients with inflammatory arthritis are not candidates for this technique as the absence of a prosthetic glenoid will result in continued glenoid erosion following humeral hemiarthroplasty. Female patients also tend to have less predictable results. This likely relates to having lower bone density and its effect on the potential for continued glenoid pain after reaming and humeral resurfacing. For male patients with osteoarthritis, the following selection criteria must be carefully considered for optimal results:

4.1 Patient factors
1.   *Age*: there are no strict age limitations. This technique is ideally suited for younger patients whose age and activity level predict glenoid failure relative to their average life expectancy. For patients older than 65 years, standard total shoulder arthroplasty is more likely to yield a predictable good to excellent result and is the preferred operation

unless patients specifically request to forgo glenoid resurfacing after discussion of the options. For the occasional older patient in this category who remains physically very active and engaged in "at risk" activities, non-prosthetic glenoid arthroplasty may be an option if other criteria are met.

2. *General Health Status*: optimal health is critical to good results after any procedure but particularly the Ream and Run. Patients with multiple comorbidities, especially those that may impair tissue healing are likely not suitable candidates for this procedure. Poorly controlled diabetes, poor nutritional status and medical problems that require the use of immunosuppressive drugs are contraindications. If there is concern about general health and nutritional status, blood work including absolute lymphocyte count (<1500 cells/mm3), serum transferrin level (<200 mg/dL) and albumin level (<3.5 g/dL) can be used to screen patients who may benefit from further optimization or consultation with a nutritionist prior to the procedure. For patients with diabetes the glycosylated hemoglobin (HgA1C) can be used to screen for glycemic control, which correlates with risk for infection and healing potential. Ideally this value should be below 7.0 for optimal healing potential. If patients are well above this mark, surgery should be delayed until their diabetes can be better controlled throughout the perioperative period

3. *Expectations*: experience has shown that recovery after this procedure generally takes longer than for a standard shoulder arthroplasty as healing of the reamed bone may progress and mature for 6 months or more and range of motion can improve for up to a year in motivated individuals. Achieving good range of motion is critical to outcomes for the Ream and Run as residual stiffness can lead to altered glenohumeral kinematics due to obligate capsular mediated translations – similar to the pathomechanics of primary shoulder osteoarthritis. Thus, patients who wish to pursue this alternative must be willing to accept a more prolonged recovery and must be sufficiently motivated to comply with the rehabilitation program including maintenance home exercises. Patients should also have exhausted all conservative measures and demonstrate sufficient pain, disability and joint degeneration to justify arthroplasty.

4. Social History:

a. *Smoking*: the dystrophic effect of smoking on tissue healing makes this a contraindication to the Ream and Run. Patients who wish to undergo this operation must be in optimal physical and nutritional health. Serum cotinine levels can be used as a method to ensure smoking cessation.

b. *History of narcotic habituation or chronic pain*: patients with a history of heavy regular use of narcotic medications are less likely to have a desirable outcome after the Ream and Run due to the potential for a more prolonged recovery process. These patients need to be appropriately counseled and advance and provisions should be made in advance of surgery to enlist a pain management specialist who can help steadily wean patients from narcotics as the healing progresses.

c. *Worker's Compensation claim or litigation*: as has been documented with many other conditions and surgeries, patients involved in a compensation claim or those litigating an injury invariably have worse outcomes after a surgical procedure. To the extent that the salvage of a failed Ream and Run requires prosthetic glenoid resurfacing, the results which are itself inferior in the revision setting, primary total shoulder arthroplasty or other surgical alternatives should be considered.

5. *Emotional History*: patients with ongoing poorly controlled mental health issues are not optimal candidates for this procedure. If patients have symptoms and disability out of proportion to the clinical scenario, have fibromyalgia or a significant poorly defined myofascial component to their pain or if patients have fallen victim to the disease construct of their condition, they are not likely to fair well with the Ream and Run procedure. The optimal patient has demonstrated a balanced self-management approach to their condition, has continued to remain active and engaged despite their physical limitation, and has demonstrated the emotional capacity to deal with the pain and life-altering nature of their diagnosis. Self-assessment scores can sometimes provide a useful window on a patient's emotional state. For instance, those patients who circle "No" on all 12 questions of the Simple Shoulder Score have a self-perceived disability that likely supersedes their actual physical limitation and their outcome after the Ream and Run will be uncertain. If a patient enters a "12" on a 0-10 Visual Analog Pain Scale, one should be concerned about the potential success of the Ream and Run.

4.2 Anatomy factors

1. *Glenoid Erosion and Morphology*: the success of Ream and Run hinges on the ability of the surgeon to achieve a smooth concavity that is oriented perpendicular to the native glenoid centerline. Preservation of subchondral bone leads to more predictable outcomes. In cases with preoperative posterior glenoid erosion, double concavity and/or posterior humeral subluxation, careful preoperative templating must be performed based on CT imaging to determine whether corrective reaming will compromise the aforementioned goals. Moderate correction often results in medialization of the glenoid, which not only reduces the surface area of the concavity but also may penetrate into the cancellous bone of the glenoid vault. In such cases, placement of a prosthetic glenoid component is recommended as hemiarthroplasty alone may result in postoperative erosion into the softer bone with consequent persistent glenoid pain. Patients noted to have decentering of the humeral head with glenoid erosion must be counseled preoperatively about the possible need for standard total shoulder arthroplasty pending the appearance of the glenoid after corrective reaming.

2. *Soft-tissue balance*: because younger patients with glenohumeral arthritis may have a variety of different arthritis types including post-traumatic and post-capsulorraphy arthropathy, there may be alteration of the soft-tissue anatomy from prior anatomy altering surgery. This is particularly the case for patients who may have undergone a prior Bristow or Latarjet type coracoid transfer in whom there can be significant scarring in the subscapularis and conjoint tendon region. If surgical releases are not able to result in a balanced soft tissue envelope that permits a wide range of motion, persistent postoperative stiffness may result in obligate translations that cause recurrent eccentric glenoid wear. Thus, a careful understanding the patients pre-operative anatomy and prior surgical history is critical to forecasting the success of the Ream and Run.

3. *Proximal humeral anatomy*: achieving an anatomical reconstruction of the proximal humerus is equally important to recentering the humeral head into a properly oriented and shaped concavity. A modern arthroplasty system that allows accurate and reliable reproduction of the native shoulder anatomy is essential and care must be taken to restore the proper relationships between the head, tuberosities and shaft in terms of the joint center of rotation and cuff insertion. A resurfacing cap may be used as an

alternative if surgeons are capable of achieving adequate glenoid exposure without humeral head osteotomy. If sequelae of prior trauma have resulted in alteration of the normal proximal humeral anatomy, specifically the head-tuberosity relationship, the surgeon must understand through appropriate imaging how this may affect the goal of achieving an anatomical reconstruction in terms of the position of the arc of the humeral convexity, center of rotation and soft-tissue balance.

5. Necessary equipment

In order to restore proper load bearing mechanics at the glenohumeral articulation, the reamed glenoid must be sufficiently concave to ensure stability, and sufficiently conforming to avoid load concentration over a small area. Thus, custom-made reamers are necessary so that there is a corresponding reamer for each humeral head diameter.(Figure 7) In order to avoid too much constraint and permit physiological glenohumeral translations, a 2mm mismatch between head diameter and reamer diameter has become the convention, as previously discussed. Thus, if the chosen head size is 52mm, a custom reamer with a diameter of curvature of 54mm is used for glenoid reaming. These reamers should enlarge in circumference as their diameter enlarges in order to contact the surface area of the native glenoid. Cannulated reamers are preferable in that they can follow a pre-drilled K-wire oriented along the glenoid centerline. This greatly improves the accuracy of the reaming process when correction is needed. An open blade reamer design is also beneficial since it allows the surgeon to see the area of bone that has been reamed during version correction.

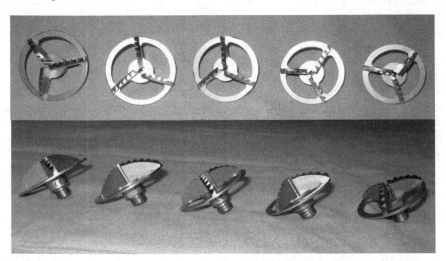

Fig. 7. Custom reamers are necessary for the Ream and Run. They should have incremental increases in the diameter of curvature by 2mm and should increase in size to cover a larger area of the glenoid face as the diameter increases. Open blade reamers are helpful in following the degree of correction during the reaming process.

An arthroplasty system of the surgeon's choice can be used with the stipulation that the chosen system allows reliable and reproducible anatomical reconstruction of proximal humeral anatomy. The author currently uses the Synthes EPOCA shoulder system (Synthes,

Westchester, PA), which includes press-fit and cemented stem options and a dual eccentricity design that allows precise placement of the humeral head on the humeral osteotomy surface. This precision improves the accuracy of restoring the humeral center of rotation and head-tuberosity relationship, which is critical in defining soft-tissue balance and proper rotator cuff function.

6. Surgical technique

The patient is positioned in a low beach chair position with the head supported in a cerebellar headrest. The body is shifted toward the operative side so the arm can be extended over the edge of the bed for humeral exposure. A rolled towel is placed beneath the medial scapular border to help orient the glenoid toward the operative field. Unless contraindicated, sterile preparation of the field should employ Choraprep solution, which has demonstrated superior bacteriocidal efficacy relative to other preparations. In addition, circumferential biodrape should be used to occlude the axillary region and cover all exposed skin. Receipt of prophylactic antibiotics must be ensured along with availability of necessary instruments and implants and confirmation of the correct patient, procedure and side.

A standard deltopectoral incision is used though some surgeons prefer a more vertical Bankart type incision in Langer's lines. The cephalic vein is taken laterally with the deltoid and the interval is developed from the clavicle to the pectoralis tendon. We do not routinely take down the pectoralis tendon unless necessary for exposure. The deltoid should be reflected off the coracoacromial ligament to facilitate exposure. The clavipectoral fascia should be excised en bloc from the inferior edge of the CA ligament superiorly to the superior edge of the pectoralis major tendon inferiorly and from the lateral border the conjoint tendon medially to the medial border of the anterior deltoid laterally. This opens the humeroscapular motion interface. A curved deltoid retractor such as a Browne's or delta Fukuda is placed behind the humeral head and a right-angle retractor such as Army Navy beneath the conjoint tendon.

The bicipital groove is opened and the biceps is sutured to the traversing pectoralis major tendon to maintain proper length and tension. It is then tenotomized in the rotator interval. The superior and inferior borders of the subscapularis are then dissected out, cauterizing or ligating the circumflex vessels. The author prefers a lesser tuberosity osteotomy for management of the subscapularis. This is done with a broad curved osteotome and started at the deepest portion of the bicipital groove. The tendon-bone fragment is tagged with suture. A curved blunt Hohman retractor is then placed along the anterior inferior humeral head and this is used to tension the humeral insertion of the inferior glenohumeral capsule-ligamentous complex. This is then released subperiosteally with progressive external rotation, and this release can be follow around to the humeral bare area posteriorly. This release greatly facilitates surgical dislocation of the humeral head.

Prior to dislocation of the humeral head, a lamina spreader type instrument can be used to distract the glenohumeral joint. This tensions the posterior capsule allowing superior visibility for thorough capsulotomy along the length of the posterior glenoid. A thorough release of the posterior capsule facilitates posterior humeral subluxation during glenoid exposure. Although some surgeons advocate selective capsular releases depending on the degree of preoperative humeral posterior subluxation, the author does not feel that capsular tissues play a role in glenohumeral stability except during the extremes of range of motion provided an adequate concavity is restored along the axis of the scapula and proper humeral retrotorsion is selected. In the author's personal series, circumferential capsular releases have never resulted in postoperative posterior instability but do improve range of motion during the early recovery. If there is a concern about posterior laxity, the rotator interval can be closed slightly more medially to provide a checkrein against posterior translation at the conclusion of the case.

The humeral osteotomy is then made along the anatomical neck generally in 25-30 degrees of retrotorsion. It is critical that this cut is flush with the articular-sided insertion of the supraspinatus tendon fibers so the anatomical reconstruction of the head-tuberosity relationship can be properly achieved.(Figure 8) Once the cut is made and refined, osteophytes around the margins of the anatomical neck can be removed, particularly those inferiorly which can cause calcar impingement with the inferior glenoid if not cleared out. A head diameter that best covers the osteotomy surface is then chosen. It is best to err toward the smaller size assuming there will be no uncovered bone that would impinge during glenohumeral rotation.

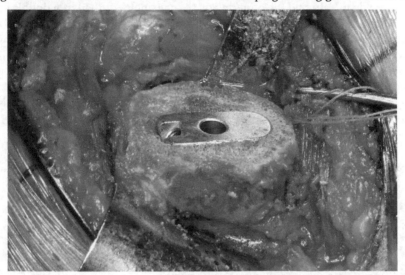

Fig. 8. The humeral osteotomy should be flush with the insertion of the supraspinatus tendon to restore the head-tuberosity relationship. The trial stem should be positioned to restore humeral retrotorsion of approximately 25-30 degrees.

If a stemmed arthroplasty is to be used, the humeral canal can then be prepped via the conventions of the given system and a trial stem placed. If a cap prosthesis is chosen, then the head can be reamed and the cap sized according to the system's technique.

The humerus is then subluxated posteriorly using a Fukuda or similar retractor. A complete circumferential release of the subscapularis can now safely be performed. The interval between the anterior capsule and inferior muscular fibers of the subscapularis is developed with Metzenbaum scissors allowing safe release of the anterior capsular from the glenoid rim and release of adhesions to the coracoid base. All adhesions should be released so that external rotation can be restored. The surgeon should feel a soft bounce when the subscapularis is pulled laterally. A blunt Hohman or spiked ribbon retractor can then be placed medially within the subscapularis fossa with the tendon and lesser tuberosity tucked medially behind it. This should allow full visualization down the anterior face of the scapular body, which is critical for restoring orientation of the glenoid concavity.

The inferior capsule is then release sharply in an extra labral fashion keeping the knife parallel to and against bone. Care should be taken to completely release the insertion of the anterior inferior and posterior inferior glenohumeral ligament from its glenoid-sided insertion. The author believes that selective capsular releases are never indicated assuming that the glenoid version is properly corrected and an adequate concavity is restored. The Fukuda retractor ring can be twisted off of the inferior glenoid rim to facilitate release of the posterior inferior capsule. Once a sufficient release has been performed, adequate glenoid exposure should permit insertion of the glenoid reamers. Internal rotation (rather than the conventional external rotation) can sometimes facilitate posterior humeral subluxation. Release of the coracohumeral ligament is sometimes necessary to improve glenoid exposure by further allowing the humerus to translate posteriorly.

The center of the existing glenoid concavity is then determined. The author uses a curved backed drill guide to help find the centering or slippage point. If there is a double concavity present, or if there is significant posterior glenoid erosion, the centering point often needs to be shifted somewhat anteriorly to properly restore glenoid version by reaming the high side. Any central ridges can be burred in advance to provisionally restore a concavity. In cases of significant posterior glenoid wear or double concavity, a flatter reamer can be used for provisional reshaping prior to definitive reestablishment of the concavity.

Once the centering point has been determined, a threaded-tipped Steinmann pin is drilled parallel to the glenoid centerline.(Figure 9) Because the scapular is a curved structure, this pin

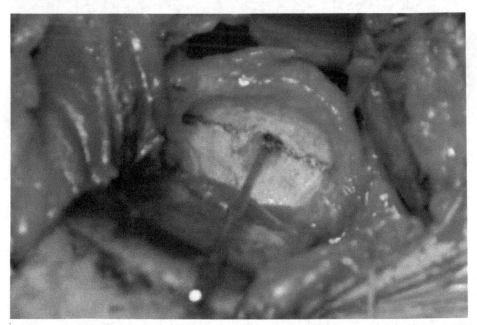

Fig. 9. The glenoid labrum is preserved during glenoid exposure and capsular releases. The centering point for the is determined and a threaded-tipped Steinmann pin is drilled to reorient the glenoid so that it is retroverted roughly 10 degrees relative to the axis of the scapular body.

should exit the anterior glenoid neck between the upper and lower crurae of the subscapularis fossa. The author uses the convention of being able to palpate the pin tip when the PIP joint of the index finger is placed against the anterior glenoid rim. If it exists too anteriorly then reaming will result in persistent retroversion that can lead to posterior instability.

Once the pin is properly positioned, the cannulated reamer can be introduced. The blades should be spinning prior to contact with the bone and the glenoid should be progressively reamed until circumferential contact occurs and a full concavity is achieved. (Figure 10) The goals of reaming are: 1) to restore glenoid version; and 2) to restore a smooth concavity. Once these goals are achieved, the surgeon must inspect the glenoid surface, the bone quality, the surface area and the degree of medialization that occurs from correction. If corrective reaming results in significant medialization, exposure of cancellous bone within the glenoid vault or loss of surface area as the glenoid narrows, placement of a glenoid prosthesis may be necessary. Ideally, there should be firm subchondral bone to support the humeral prosthesis.

Next a small drill is used to make multiple perforations in the reamed glenoid face. This serves two purposes.(Figure 11) Firstly, it decompresses the venous congestion than can occur in arthritic bone, which may improve pain relief. Secondly, it permits egress of bone marrow stem cells to help reform a fibro-cartilaginous coating on the reamed glenoid face.

The final humeral prosthesis is then inserted according to the specifications of the system. It is critical that the humeral head be optimally positioned to restore the center of rotation of the joint and to restore the proper head-tuberosity relationship.(Figure 12)

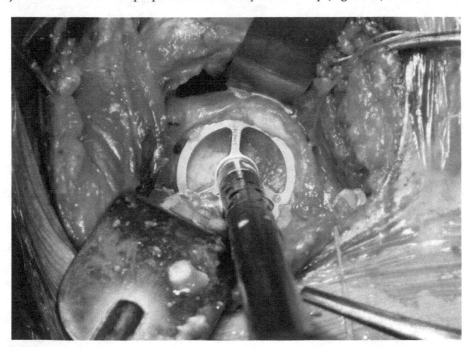

Fig. 10. The chosen reamer is introduced and the glenoid reamed until a smooth concavity is achieved.

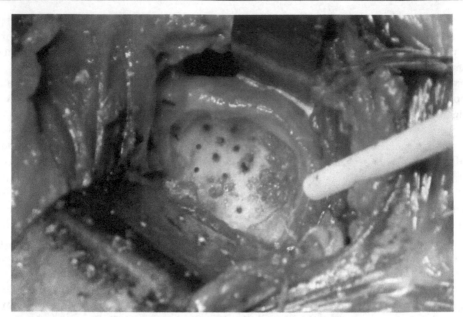

Fig. 11. Multiple holes are drilled into the reamed glenoid to decompress venous congestion and promote egress of stem cells to promote fibrocartilage formation.

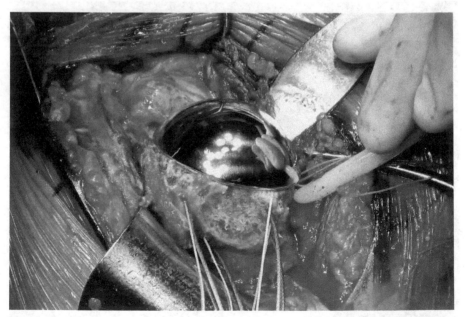

Fig. 12. The humeral head must achieve anatomical reconstruction with regard to coverage of the osteotomy and restoration of the head-shaft and head-tuberosity relationship. The head should have an anatomical height that does not overstuff the joint.

Excess anterior and posterior overhang must be avoided and there should be smooth transition at the calcar that prevents boney impingement in this region. A head thickness that corresponds to normal anatomy should be chosen. If the system used provides 3 offset options for each diameter, it is best to choose the middle size to prevent over or under stuffing of the joint. Conventional on-table measurements of passive translation are not helpful in determining proper soft tissue tension as they do no correlate with dynamic stability in the mid range of motion after surgery. It is best to err toward the looser side with the Ream and Run as it facilitates recovery of motion which is critical to outcomes and it does not correlate with postoperative instability assuming the glenoid has been properly corrected.

A secure subscapularis repair is essential to permit early range of motion. The author currently uses the technique described by Millett et al using cerclage sutures looped around the humeral stem.[47] If a porous ingrowth stem is used, the author uses two 1mm cables instead because micromotion of the sutures against the stem coating will result in suture rupture.(Figure 13) These cables are supplemented by a suture tension band construct tied over a cortical button lateral to the bicipital groove. If cables are used, the crimps are positioned in the bicipital groove and covered over by the biceps tendon to prevent soft-tissue irritation. The lateral part of the rotator interval is then closed. If there is concern about posterior instability, additional interval sutures can be placed more medially though this may compromise external rotation and potentially decentralize the humeral head.

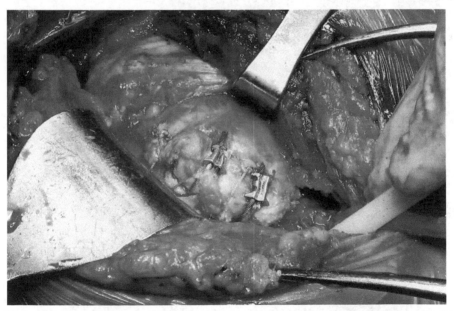

Fig. 13. A secure repair of the subscapularis is essential regardless of the technique. In this picture, horizontal cerclage cables have been used to compress the lesser tuberosity fragment to its osteotomy bed.

7. Post-operative protocol

Immediate range of motion exercises are begun under the supervision of the therapist. Forward elevation to 140 degree and external rotation to 40 degree is allowed along with external rotation isometrics, scapular pinches and cervical and elbow range of motion. Patients are instructed on how to perform active-assisted range of motion exercises and encouraged to do so several times daily. Positional exercises, such as placing the arm on the rest of a couch are also permitted. This holds a static position of stretch for a period of time that does not jeopardize the repair. Most patients are discharged from the hospital with home services and transition to outpatient therapy after their first postoperative visit around 10-14 days.

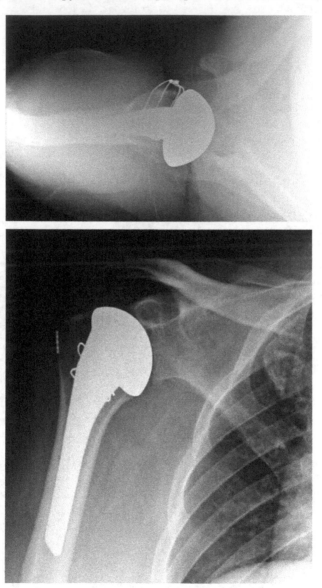

Fig. 14. A and B: Postoperative AP and axillary lateral radiographs demonstrating anatomical reconstruction of the humerus with creation of a smooth concavity.

Around 4 weeks, progressive return to maximal range of motion is permitted and exercises such as wall walks can be added. Active internal rotation is discouraged to protect the subscapularis. Patients are instructed to still limit use of the arm for physical activities and focus on flexibility.

At 8 weeks, the focus continues on maximizing range of motion. The subscapularis repair must still be protected from active internal rotation but patients can begin some posterior capsular stretching and light deltoid, trapezius and periscapular strengthening.

Assuming adequate progress and a negative belly-press test at 12 weeks, patients can start internal rotation strengthening and progressive use of the arm for normal daily activities. Return to physically demanding activities and sports requires at least 4 or more months to ensure and adequately healed subscapularis

In the author's experience in trying to accelerate the rehabilitation protocol, the subscapularis must be protected at all costs. Rupture can occur all the way out to three months despite what appears to be a very durable repair at the time of surgery. Rupture tends to occur from overzealous therapy or patient non-compliance and thus both parties must be educated about realistic goals and expectations during the early recovery.

By six months after surgery a full range of activities are permitted as tolerated by the patient's comfort and demands. Given the absence of concern about failure of a prosthetic glenoid, no specific restrictions are placed on patients activities. Maintenance stretching and strengthening exercises are strongly encouraged for up to 2 years as pain relief, motion and function see to go hand-in-hand in their potential to improve throughout this prolonged interval.

8. Complications

Complications of shoulder arthroplasty are well-documented and the Ream and Run is no exception to the conventional and well-accepted adversities that can occur from any open shoulder surgery such as infection and axillary nerve injury. The following discussion will focus on complications that are particularly pertinent though not exclusive to the Ream and Run procedure.

8.1 Glenoid wear and erosion

As has been previously discussed, overzealous reaming or the need for excessive glenoid version correction can result in penetration of the subchondral plate and exposure of cancellous bone in the glenoid vault. It can also result in narrowing of the anterior-posterior dimensions of the glenoid concavity, which reduces the overall surface area for contact stress distribution and predisposes to instability. In these situations, patients will continue to experience pain following humeral hemiarthroplasty and may demonstrate recurrent glenoid erosion both medially and posteriorly. Thus patient selection and work-up are critical to predicting who is the ideal candidate likely to have a good outcome and all patients must be counseled about the potential need for glenoid replacement if the principles and goals of non-prosthetic glenoid arthroplasty cannot be met intraoperatively. Rhee and colleagues have shown that the results of salvage glenoid replacement after failed hemiarthroplasty are inferior to primary total shoulder arthroplasty.[48] This highlights the importance of doing the right operation the first time around.

8.2 Subscapularis rupture

Despite the added security afforded by lesser tuberosity osteotomy, failure can still occur if undue stress is placed on the repair. While the contention maintains that lesser tuberosity osteotomy allows bone to bone healing, this is not guaranteed in all cases. Micromotion at the repair site may stimulate a fibrous union, and release of the subscapularis intraoperatively may disrupt the blood supply to this fragment resulting in avascular necrosis of the lesser tuberosity and inability to heal directly by bony union. While this has not been previously reported in the literature, the author has had occasion to explore 4 cases in which the lesser tuberosity repair ruptured after surgery as detected clinically and radiographically. In all cases, the bone was sclerotic and devoid of any bleeding when drilled at the time of re-repair. Future studies will need to better determine the biology of lesser tuberosity healing but until more is known about how to optimize this process, erring on the side of caution is the safest route to avoid the devastating complication of subscapularis failure. This fact is true regardless of the method of tendon repair used. Because these patients tend to be more active and aggressive in terms of lifestyle pursuits, they need to be educated in terms of recovery expectations so that their ambitions do not compromise their compliance with the recovery protocol.

8.3 Stiffness
Recovery of range of motion is critical to outcomes after the Ream and Run procedure. Residual stiffness will result in obligate, capsular-mediated translations that equate to the same pathomechanics resulting in posterior humeral subluxation and glenoid erosion. The author believes that in all cases, aggressive circumferential capsular releases are necessary to restore motion and selective releases for fear of instability are never indicated. Capsular-mediated stability only occurs at the terminal range of motion, which is never a concern in the first 3 months after surgery when the capsule is reforming around the prosthetic joint. Stability in the mid-range is a function of a properly oriented glenoid concavity of sufficient area and a functional rotator cuff. Surgeons should not rely on intraoperative tests of joint stability that measure capsular tension as they are largely irrelevant assuming a properly performed reconstruction.

Given the prior discussion about subscapularis failure, range of motion exercises must be a graduated process that focuses more on frequency than exertion for the first several weeks. Patients must take an active but responsible and educated role in their own recovery and they must understand the potential consequences of noncompliance. This is a delicate balance that requires pre and postoperative education from both the surgeon and therapist. The author has also found it invaluable to identify one or two therapists who take an interest in shoulder arthroplasty and have a better understanding of how to achieve desired results. As with any discipline, frequency, volume and practice beget experience and results in this regard.

9. Results

When patient selection is combined with surgical technique that achieves the principles of Ream and Run, outcomes can be comparable to total shoulder arthroplasty in terms of pain relief, range of motion and function. Given that no specific restrictions are placed on patients postoperatively, results in terms of return to physically demanding leisure time physical activities can be outstanding. Patients have returned to sports such as water skiing, weight lifting, competitive tennis, and other outdoor pursuits. As many of these patients previously engaged in activities that may have contributed to early glenohumeral degenerative disease, the ability to return to similar activities, albeit in a modified setting, is a significant improvement in their health-related quality of life.

The author currently performs the Ream and Run procedures in roughly 8% of all arthroplasty cases. Generally, it is reserved for male patients aged 65 or less who meet the criteria previously discussed and who understand and accept the longer recovery in favor of the absence of restrictions. Between 2004-2010, 55 Ream and Run cases have been performed in 52 patients ranging in age from 42-68 years (average 56 years). This series has included 50 males and 2 females. Although formal outcome measures have not been performed on this consecutive series, 5 patients have required additional surgery. Two patients underwent revision glenoid resurfacing for recalcitrant pain with recurrent posterior erosion at 16 and 26 months after the index procedure. One of these patients was female. The other was subsequently determined to have inflammatory osteoarthritis. Two patients underwent repair of a partial subscapularis rupture both of whom were noted to have a smooth, remodeled concavity with rests of fibrocartilage at the time of exploration 3 and 47 months postoperatively. One patient underwent explantation of the humeral prosthesis due to deep infection with Staph. Epidermidis. This patient was subsequently revised to a standard total shoulder arthroplasty after interval placement of an antibiotic cement spacer and parenteral antimicrobial treatment. Two additional patients have complained of persistent pain but have elected not to undergo further surgery. Neither of these patients has demonstrated significant glenoid erosion to suggest that the cause of pain is in fact due to wear at the articulation.

Lynch et al have reported on outcomes of the Ream and Run procedure at mid-term follow-up. In the initial report, 32 of 35 patients demonstrated improved function regaining an average of 4.5 functions on the Simple Shoulder Test (SST).[49] Overall average SST score improved from 4.7 to 9.4 at 2-4 years follow-up. Sequential improvement in function was noted all the way up to 36 months after surgery. Patients who had radiographic evidence of a joint space on postoperative x-rays had better outcomes indicating that presumed formation of a fibrocartilage interface correlates with better pain relief and improvement in function. Clinton et al in a similar series demonstrated outcomes comparable to a matched set of patients undergoing total shoulder arthroplasty.[50] Again, functional outcomes for those patients undergoing the Ream and Run were noted to improve sequentially out to 3 years postoperatively.

Recently, Saltzman et al reported on outcomes of the Ream and Run in patients aged 55 years or younger. In terms of pre versus postoperative comparative SST, 53 of 56 patients were improved to a degree comparable to patients who underwent a total shoulder arthroplasty by the same surgeon.[51] Patients with mild preoperative glenoid erosion did not demonstrate progression while one patient with moderate erosion progressed to severe erosion. Average medial glenoid erosion measured 1.1 mm at an average of 44 months with the worst case measuring 6.3mm. Nine of 65 shoulders required revision including 4 (6%) conversions to a total shoulder for painful glenoid wear. Patients who underwent revision surgery tended to have a more complicated preoperative course including more severe functional deficits to overcome and a higher incidence of multiple prior surgeries.

Collectively, these results are comparable or superior to previously discussed literature looking at hemiarthroplasty alone or biological resurfacing techniques in this age cohort.[23, 25, 29, 33, 52] As our experience with this technique grows, patient selection criteria, indications and techniques have been refined to reflect potential modes of failure and their risk factors. As with all of orthopedics, the right operation for the right problem in the right patient is the key to success. The shoulder arthroplasty surgeon must carefully evaluate each candidate clinically, radiographically and in terms of compliance and expectations. When proper surgical technique is applied to right clinical setting the results of the Ream and Run can be both impressive and lasting and should be a tool in the shoulder surgeons armamentarium for management of advanced arthritis in the young and active patient.

10. References

[1] Farron A, Terrier A, Buchler P. Risks of loosening of a prosthetic glenoid implanted in retroversion. *J Shoulder Elbow Surg*. 2006;15:521-526.

[2] Oosterom R, Rozing PM, Verdonschot N, Bersee HE. Effect of joint conformity on glenoid component fixation in total shoulder arthroplasty. *Proc Inst Mech Eng H*. 2004;218:339-347.

[3] Hopkins AR, Hansen UN, Amis AA et al. Wear in the prosthetic shoulder: association with design parameters. *J Biomech Eng*. 2007;129:223-230.

[4] Braman JP, Falicov A, Boorman R, Matsen FAr. Alterations in surface geometry in retrieved polyethylene glenoid component. *J Orthop Res*. 2006;24:1249-1260.

[5] Hertel R, Ballmer FT. Observations on retrieved glenoid components. *J Arthroplasty*. 2003;18:361-366.

[6] Nho SJ, Nam D, Ala OL, Craig EV, Warren RF, Wright TM. Observations on retrieved glenoid components from total shoulder arthroplasty. *J Shoulder Elbow Surg*. 2009;18:371-378.

[7] Arnold RM, High RR, Grosshans KT, Walker CW, Fehringer EV. Bone presence between the central peg's radial fins of a partially cemented pegged all poly glenoid component suggest few radiolucencies. *J Shoulder Elbow Surg*. 2011;20:315-321.

[8] Barwood S, Setter KJ, Blaine TA, Bigliani LU. The incidence of early radiolucencies about a pegged glenoid component using cement pressurization. *J Shoulder Elbow Surg*. 2008;17:703-708.

[9] Churchill RS, Zellmer C, Zimmers HJ, Ruggero R. Clinical and radiographic analysis of a partially cemented glenoid implant: five-year minimum follow-up. *J Shoulder Elbow Surg*. 2010;19:1091-1097.

[10] Groh GI. Survival and radiographic analysis of a glenoid component with a cementless fluted central peg. *J Shoulder Elbow Surg*. 2010;19:1265-1268.

[11] Walch G, Young AA, Melis B, Gazielly D, Loew M, Boileau P. Results of a convex-back cemented keeled glenoid component in primary osteoarthritis: multicenter study with a follow-up greater than 5 years. *J Shoulder Elbow Surg*. 2011;20:385-394.

[12] Young A, Walch G, Boileau P et al. A multicentre study of the long-term results of using a flat-back polyethylene glenoid component in shoulder replacement for primary osteoarthritis. *J Bone Joint Surg Br*. 2011;93:210-216.

[13] Kasten P, Pape G, Raiss P et al. Mid-term survivorship analysis of a shoulder replacement with a keeled glenoid and a modern cementing technique. *J Bone Joint Surg Br*. 2010;92:387-392.

[14] Bartelt R, Sperling JW, Schleck CD, Cofield RH. Shoulder arthroplasty in patients aged fifty-five years or younger with osteoarthritis. *J Shoulder Elbow Surg*. 2011;20:123-130.

[15] Fox TJ, Cil A, Sperling JW, Sanchez-Sotelo J, Schleck CD, Cofield RH. Survival of the glenoid component in shoulder arthroplasty. *J Shoulder Elbow Surg*. 2009;18:859-863.

[16] Taunton MJ, McIntosh AL, Sperling JW, Cofield RH. Total shoulder arthroplasty with a metal-backed, bone-ingrowth glenoid component. Medium to long-term results. *J Bone Joint Surg Am*. 2008;90:2180-2188.

[17] Tammachote N, Sperling JW, Vathana T, Cofield RH, Harmsen WS, Schleck CD. Long-term results of cemented metal-backed glenoid components for osteoarthritis of the shoulder. *J Bone Joint Surg Am*. 2009;91:160-166.

[18] Boileau P, Avidor C, Krishnan SG, Walch G, Kempf JF, Mole D. Cemented polyethylene versus uncemented metal-backed glenoid components in total shoulder arthroplasty: a prospective, double-blind, randomized study. *J Shoulder Elbow Surg.* 2002;11:351-359.

[19] Cheung EV, Sperling JW, Cofield RH. Reimplantation of a glenoid component following component removal and allogenic bone-grafting. *J Bone Joint Surg Am.* 2007;89:1777-1783.

[20] Cheung EV, Sperling JW, Cofield RH. Revision shoulder arthroplasty for glenoid component loosening. *J Shoulder Elbow Surg.* 2008;17:371-375.

[21] Neyton L, Walch G, Nove-Josserand L, Edwards TB. Glenoid corticocancellous bone grafting after glenoid component removal in the treatment of glenoid loosening. *J Shoulder Elbow Surg.* 2006;15:173-179.

[22] Phipatanakul WP, Norris TR. Treatment of glenoid loosening and bone loss due to osteolysis with glenoid bone grafting. *J Shoulder Elbow Surg.* 2006;15:84-87.

[23] Burkhead WZJ, Hutton KS. Biologic resurfacing of the glenoid with hemiarthroplasty of the shoulder. *J Shoulder Elbow Surg.* 1995;4:263-270.

[24] Burkhead WZJ, Krishnan SG, Lin KC. Biologic resurfacing of the arthritic glenohumeral joint: Historical review and current applications. *J Shoulder Elbow Surg.* 2007;16:S248-53.

[25] Elhassan B, Ozbaydar M, Diller D, Higgins LD, Warner JJ. Soft-tissue resurfacing of the glenoid in the treatment of glenohumeral arthritis in active patients less than fifty years old. *J Bone Joint Surg Am.* 2009;91:419-424.

[26] Lee KT, Bell S, Salmon J. Cementless surface replacement arthroplasty of the shoulder with biologic resurfacing of the glenoid. *J Shoulder Elbow Surg.* 2009;18:915-919.

[27] Wirth MA. Humeral head arthroplasty and meniscal allograft resurfacing of the glenoid. *J Bone Joint Surg Am.* 2009;91:1109-1119.

[28] Nicholson GP, Goldstein JL, Romeo AA et al. Lateral meniscus allograft biologic glenoid arthroplasty in total shoulder arthroplasty for young shoulders with degenerative joint disease. *J Shoulder Elbow Surg.* 2007;16:S261-6.

[29] de Beer JF, Bhatia DN, van Rooyen KS, Du Toit DF. Arthroscopic debridement and biological resurfacing of the glenoid in glenohumeral arthritis. *Knee Surg Sports Traumatol Arthrosc.* 2010;18:1767-1773.

[30] Savoie FHr, Brislin KJ, Argo D. Arthroscopic glenoid resurfacing as a surgical treatment for glenohumeral arthritis in the young patient: midterm results. *Arthroscopy.* 2009;25:864-871.

[31] Gerber C, Snedeker JG, Krause AS, Appenzeller A, Farshad M. Osteochondral glenoid allograft for biologic resurfacing of the glenoid: biomechanical comparison of novel design concepts. *J Shoulder Elbow Surg.* 2011

[32] Bryant D, Litchfield R, Sandow M, Gartsman GM, Guyatt G, Kirkley A. A comparison of pain, strength, range of motion, and functional outcomes after hemiarthroplasty and total shoulder arthroplasty in patients with osteoarthritis of the shoulder. A systematic review and meta-analysis. *J Bone Joint Surg Am.* 2005;87:1947-1956.

[33] Sperling JW, Cofield RH, Rowland CM. Minimum fifteen-year follow-up of Neer hemiarthroplasty and total shoulder arthroplasty in patients aged fifty years or younger. *J Shoulder Elbow Surg.* 2004;13:604-613.

[34] Edwards TB, Kadakia NR, Boulahia A et al. A comparison of hemiarthroplasty and total shoulder arthroplasty in the treatment of primary glenohumeral osteoarthritis: results of a multicenter study. *J Shoulder Elbow Surg.* 2003;12:207-213.

[35] Lo IK, Litchfield RB, Griffin S, Faber K, Patterson SD, Kirkley A. Quality-of-life outcome following hemiarthroplasty or total shoulder arthroplasty in patients with osteoarthritis. A prospective, randomized trial. *J Bone Joint Surg Am*. 2005;87:2178-2185.

[36] Levine WN, Djurasovic M, Glasson JM, Pollock RG, Flatow EL, Bigliani LU. Hemiarthroplasty for glenohumeral osteoarthritis: results correlated to degree of glenoid wear. *J Shoulder Elbow Surg*. 1997;6:449-454.

[37] Matsen FAr, Clinton J, Lynch J, Bertelsen A, Richardson ML. Glenoid component failure in total shoulder arthroplasty. *J Bone Joint Surg Am*. 2008;90:885-896.

[38] Milgram JW, Rana NA. Pathologic evaluation of the failed cup arthroplasty: a review of 32 cases. *Clin Orthop Relat Res*. 1981;158-179.

[39] Milgram JW, Rana NA. Roentgenologic and clinical evaluation of vitallium mold arthroplasty of the hip. *Surg Gynecol Obstet*. 1968;127:1042-1050.

[40] Enneking WF, Singsen ET. Pathologic changes in the idiopathic painful cup arthroplasty. *Clin Orthop Relat Res*. 1974;236-253.

[41] D'Ambrosia RD, McClain EJ, Wissinger HA, Riggins RS. Resorption of the femoral head beneath the vitallium mold. *Surg Forum*. 1972;23:465-467.

[42] Weldon EJr, Boorman RS, Smith KL, Matsen FAr. Optimizing the glenoid contribution to the stability of a humeral hemiarthroplasty without a prosthetic glenoid. *J Bone Joint Surg Am*. 2004;86-A:2022-2029.

[43] Matsen FAr, Clark JM, Titelman RM et al. Healing of reamed glenoid bone articulating with a metal humeral hemiarthroplasty: a canine model. *J Orthop Res*. 2005;23:18-26.

[44] Clinton J, Warme WJ, Lynch JR, Lippitt SB, Matsen FAr. Shoulder hemiarthroplasty with nonprosthetic glenoid arthroplasty: The Ream and Run. *Techniques in Shoulder and Elbow Surgery*. 2009;10:43-52.

[45] Pearl ML, Kurutz S. Geometric analysis of commonly used prosthetic systems for proximal humeral replacement. *J Bone Joint Surg Am*. 1999;81:660-671.

[46] Pearl ML, Kurutz S, Postachini R. Geometric variables in anatomic replacement of the proximal humerus: how much prosthetic geometry is necessary? *J Shoulder Elbow Surg*. 2009;18:366-370.

[47] Ponce BA, Ahluwalia RS, Mazzocca AD, Gobezie RG, Warner JJ, Millett PJ. Biomechanical and clinical evaluation of a novel lesser tuberosity repair technique in total shoulder arthroplasty. *J Bone Joint Surg Am*. 2005;87 Suppl 2:1-8.

[48] Rhee PC, Sassoon AA, Schleck CD, Harmsen WS, Sperling JW, Cofield RH. Revision total shoulder arthroplasty for painful glenoid arthrosis after humeral head replacement: the posttraumatic shoulder. *J Shoulder Elbow Surg*. 2011

[49] Lynch JR, Franta AK, Montgomery WHJ, Lenters TR, Mounce D, Matsen FAr. Self-assessed outcome at two to four years after shoulder hemiarthroplasty with concentric glenoid reaming. *J Bone Joint Surg Am*. 2007;89:1284-1292.

[50] Clinton J, Franta AK, Lenters TR, Mounce D, Matsen FAr. Nonprosthetic glenoid arthroplasty with humeral hemiarthroplasty and total shoulder arthroplasty yield similar self-assessed outcomes in the management of comparable patients with glenohumeral arthritis. *J Shoulder Elbow Surg*. 2007;16:534-538.

[51] Saltzman MD, Chamberlain AM, Mercer DM, Warme WJ, Bertelsen AL, Matsen FAr. Shoulder hemiarthroplasty with concentric glenoid reaming in patients 55 years old or less. *J Shoulder Elbow Surg*. 2011;20:609-615.

[52] Krishnan SG, Reineck JR, Nowinski RJ, Harrison D, Burkhead WZ. Humeral hemiarthroplasty with biologic resurfacing of the glenoid for glenohumeral arthritis. Surgical technique. *J Bone Joint Surg Am*. 2008;90 Suppl 2 Pt 1:9-19.

Permissions

The contributors of this book come from diverse backgrounds, making this book a truly international effort. This book will bring forth new frontiers with its revolutionizing research information and detailed analysis of the nascent developments around the world.

We would like to thank Dr. Samo K. Fokter, MD, for lending his expertise to make the book truly unique. He has played a crucial role in the development of this book. Without his invaluable contribution this book wouldn't have been possible. He has made vital efforts to compile up to date information on the varied aspects of this subject to make this book a valuable addition to the collection of many professionals and students.

This book was conceptualized with the vision of imparting up-to-date information and advanced data in this field. To ensure the same, a matchless editorial board was set up. Every individual on the board went through rigorous rounds of assessment to prove their worth. After which they invested a large part of their time researching and compiling the most relevant data for our readers. Conferences and sessions were held from time to time between the editorial board and the contributing authors to present the data in the most comprehensible form. The editorial team has worked tirelessly to provide valuable and valid information to help people across the globe.

Every chapter published in this book has been scrutinized by our experts. Their significance has been extensively debated. The topics covered herein carry significant findings which will fuel the growth of the discipline. They may even be implemented as practical applications or may be referred to as a beginning point for another development. Chapters in this book were first published by InTech; hereby published with permission under the Creative Commons Attribution License or equivalent.

The editorial board has been involved in producing this book since its inception. They have spent rigorous hours researching and exploring the diverse topics which have resulted in the successful publishing of this book. They have passed on their knowledge of decades through this book. To expedite this challenging task, the publisher supported the team at every step. A small team of assistant editors was also appointed to further simplify the editing procedure and attain best results for the readers.

Our editorial team has been hand-picked from every corner of the world. Their multi-ethnicity adds dynamic inputs to the discussions which result in innovative outcomes. These outcomes are then further discussed with the researchers and contributors who give their valuable feedback and opinion regarding the same. The feedback is then collaborated with the researches and they are edited in a comprehensive manner to aid the understanding of the subject.

Apart from the editorial board, the designing team has also invested a significant amount of their time in understanding the subject and creating the most relevant covers. They scrutinized every image to scout for the most suitable representation of the subject and create an appropriate cover for the book.

The publishing team has been involved in this book since its early stages. They were actively engaged in every process, be it collecting the data, connecting with the contributors or procuring relevant information. The team has been an ardent support to the editorial, designing and production team. Their endless efforts to recruit the best for this project, has resulted in the accomplishment of this book. They are a veteran in the field of academics and their pool of knowledge is as vast as their experience in printing. Their expertise and guidance has proved useful at every step. Their uncompromising quality standards have made this book an exceptional effort. Their encouragement from time to time has been an inspiration for everyone.

The publisher and the editorial board hope that this book will prove to be a valuable piece of knowledge for researchers, students, practitioners and scholars across the globe.

List of Contributors

Peter Schäfer and Dieter Sandow
MVZ Labor Ludwigsburg, Wernerstrasse 33, Ludwigsburg, Germany

Lars Frommelt
Institute for Infectiology, ENDO-Clinic Hamburg, Holstenstrasse 2, Hamburg, Germany

Bernd Fink
Department of Joint Replacement, General and Rheumatic Orthopaedics, Orthopaedic Clinic Markgröningen, Kurt-Lindemann-Weg 10, Markgröningen, Germany

Michelle M. Dowsey, Trisha N. Peel and Peter F.M. Choong
University of Melbourne, Department of Surgery, St. Vincent's Hospital Melbourne, Department of Orthopaedics, St. Vincent's Hospital Melbourne, Australia

Weisheng Ye, Wei Shang and Yaqiong Yang
Tianjin Orthopaedics Hospital, P. R. China

J. Bahebeck, D. Handy Eone, B. Ngo Nonga and T. Kingue Njie
University Hospitals of Yaoundé, Cameroon

Fred H. Geisler
Chicago Back Institute, Swedish Covenant Hospital, N. Francisco, Chicago, IL, USA

Bruce V. Darden
OrthoCarolina Spine Center, Charlotte, USA

José Hernández Enríquez, Xavier A. Duralde and Antonio J. Pérez Caballer
Orthopaedics Department, Hospital Infanta Elena, Valdemoro, Spain
Orthopaedics Department, Peachtree Orthopaedic Clinic, Atlanta GA, USA
Orthopaedics Department, Hospital Infanta Elena, Valdemoro, Spain

Nicola Massy-Westropp
School of Health Sciences, University of South Australia, Australia

Michael W. Maier
Department of Orthopedics, Trauma Surgery and Paraplegiology, University of Heidelberg, Heidelberg, Germany

Philip Kasten
Carl-Gustav Carus University of Dresden, Dresden, Germany

Moby Parsons
Seacoast Orthopedics and Sports Medicine, Somersworth, NH, USA